Praise for
Real Love for I

"When the harsh winds of life break th
competency, I long for a heart that bur
warm and inviting. Andi Ashworth has such a heart and welcomes us to a
hearth where we find comfort and courage. Her words in *Real Love for
Real Life* offer us a taste of the kindness of Jesus. Page by page you will find
your burdens less difficult to bear. Even more remarkable, you will be drawn
to the glorious desire to offer a safe harbor to others. I will be drawn to
re-read this book often to know what it is to care and to be well cared for."

—DAN B. ALLENDER, president of Mars Hill Graduate School
and author of *The Wounded Heart* and *The Healing Path*

"Andi inspires us as she reminds us that there are no mundane moments
in our lives. Reading this book makes me wish I were in her family or were
one of the cherished friends who gets to feast on the richness of relationship with her!"

—KIM HILL, recording artist and musician

"Caregivers who have often felt unimportant or insignificant will breathe
out *amens* as they read about how God values their gifts of hospitality
and creative home building. *Real Love for Real Life* will also open the eyes and
challenge the hearts of those who are unaware of the life of sacrifice that
caregivers lead."

—KIM THOMAS, author of *Simplicity: Finding Peace
by Uncluttering Your Life* and *Living in the Sacred Now*

"*Real Love for Real Life* is the most original book we've read in years. Andi
encourages, inspires, challenges, and dignifies the caregiver. With wisdom
and grace she offers a vision of a life lived with true purpose and hope.
Real Love for Real Life will change the way your family lives."

—KATIE AND DAN HASELTINE, Jars of Clay

REAL LOVE
for
REAL *Life*

REAL LOVE
for
REAL *Life*

The Art and Work
of Caring

Andi Ashworth

SHAW BOOKS
an imprint of WATERBROOK PRESS

Real Love for Real Life
A SHAW BOOK
PUBLISHED BY WATERBROOK PRESS
2375 Telstar Drive, Suite 160
Colorado Springs, Colorado 80920
A division of Random House, Inc.

All Scripture quotations, unless otherwise indicated, are taken from the *Holy Bible, New International Version*®. NIV®. Copyright © 1973, 1978, 1984 by International Bible Society. Used by permission of Zondervan Publishing House. All rights reserved. Scripture quotations also taken from the *New American Standard Bible*® (NASB). © Copyright The Lockman Foundation 1960, 1962, 1963, 1968, 1971, 1972, 1973, 1975, 1977, 1995. Used by permission (www. Lockman.org).

ISBN 0-87788-048-4

Printed in the United States of America
2002—First Edition

10 9 8 7 6 5 4 3 2 1

Dedicated to
my mother,
Marilyn Jeanne Ickes, 1930–1984,
and my grandmother,
Martha Frances McKee, 1901–1977

CONTENTS

ACKNOWLEDGMENTS

Vocations are often discovered in the company of those who help name us. I have a special gratitude for those who encouraged me over the years to write and who gave me the name "writer": Chuck (my husband), Judi Daniels, Paula Williams, Bruce McCurdy, and Barbara Haynes.

I'm deeply grateful to my best friend, Maggie Anthony, who kept reminding me of my calling to this topic. Thank you, Maggie, for the daffodils on my first day of writing, for the meals and the warm bed whenever I need them, for asking, listening, praying, and nurturing. Thank you, Betty Gilpin, for our years of conversations about the themes in this book. A special thanks to Virginia Bousquet, whose faithfulness as a praying friend is an invaluable gift. Thank you to Marty Briner and the late Bob Briner, for always asking, "Are you writing?" Thank you to my mother-in-law, Alice Ashworth, for your love and encouragement, and for modeling a life of caring.

I'm grateful to Karen Crowe, Jody Barker, and Linda Preston for making important contributions to this book through e-mail conversations. Thank you for being willing to share your stories. To my dear friends Kathi Smith, Judi Daniels, and Diana Beach, and my sister, Laurie Woods—I'm thankful for your valuable input.

A world of thanks to the pastoral couples who've been so faithful to teach and care for our family over the years: John and Laura Cowan, Mary and Louis Neely, Scotty and Darlene Smith, Mike and Rinda Smith, and Scott and Linda Roley. Eternal gratitude to Mike and Julie Butera for welcoming us into the kingdom.

To Don Pape and Elisa Fryling Stanford—thank you for embracing me and for giving this book a chance to come to life. Elisa, I'm so grateful for your amazing editorial gifts. And your gentle encouragement saw me through every step of the writing process. Don, thank you for cheering me on with words and prayers. I can't imagine a better experience for a first-time author than the one I've had with you two. Your friendship has been the icing on the cake!

Thank you to my oldest group of friends from whom I learned early in life about the joys of women's friendship: Joanne Devine, Jenae Meford, and Lynne Lyle.

A very special thank-you to Edith Schaeffer and Susan Schaeffer Macaulay. I am forever grateful to you both for being voices of sanity, help, and inspiration through your books and audiotapes. To the L'Abri Fellowship worldwide—your work is extremely important. Press on!

To my sister, Paula Williams—your love and encouragement are never ending. Thank you for always showing an interest, always listening, for reading early chapters, for your confidence in me, and your input into the book. Your voice is a constant comfort.

To my daughter and son-in-law, Molly and Mark Nicholas, and my son and daughter-in-law, Sam and Meg Ashworth—I love you *so* much. Thank you for being proud of me, for your appreciation, your encouragement, your prayers. This book is for you. And Mark, thanks for the photos!

To Chuck—my greatest advocate. You've given me unending help and support, beginning with my first inclination to write on this topic. You've never wavered in your confidence in me and your belief in the importance of this book. I've leaned on you in so many ways—thank you for taking care of me. My gratitude runs deep. I love you.

EMBRACING THE TRUTH
ABOUT CAREGIVING

Sometimes you find meaning, purpose, and good in the most unexpected places. Without intending to, I entered a vocation I had previously stereotyped, misunderstood, and demeaned. I became a mother and a homemaker. It was my entrance into a life with many doors and passageways, each leading to the art and work of caring for people on a thousand fronts.

I've come to understand this caring work as a calling, one that continues to beckon even now that my children are grown. Seasons of life bring new incarnations, but caregiving remains a vital part of who I am. It's not that I haven't struggled with some of the work or grown weary of feeling invisible to the world. I have. But more significantly, I've been captured by the truth that my life and work change the shape of people and their worlds. This makes it important work. And because it has such power, I take it very seriously.

Early on, I discovered that, with design, intent, and hard work, I could contribute to a story laced with the true, the good, and the beautiful in the lives of my friends and family. With millions of other coworkers, I've embraced the truth that we, as children of a creative God, are called to recover and practice the art of caregiving.

Most of us have an image in our minds when we think of caregiving. We get our ideas from different sources—society, our families, the Church. Perhaps we think of a nurse, a home-health aide, or a hospice worker. While these are all true descriptions of a caregiver, caregiving is a much larger reality that encompasses a broad spectrum of relationships over a lifetime. Though caregivers can be paid professionals, *unpaid* caregiving work—work fundamental to sustaining the human race—takes place every day in the corners and pockets and glaringly obvious places of our world.

The nitty-gritty work of caring for human life is mainly behind the scenes, quiet, and matter-of-fact. As a result, caregiving is often taken for granted; no one realizes it is the result of someone's work. I've come to realize that the only people who really know about caregiving are the ones engaged in it or experienced with it—and even they do not always know how to fully express what their vocation is because they're not used to considering it as real, dignified work.

Real Love for Real Life was born out of my own need to gain a fuller understanding of what it means to give care. In particular seasons of caregiving, I've looked for help to address the complexities of my day-to-day life. Sadly, few of the books I read and little of the teaching I received offered such help. When caregiving was mentioned at all, it was often patronized or sentimentalized. At other times it was dismissed or ignored completely. On rare occasions, I came across an author or another person who actually understood the realities of my daily work and spoke of it with respect. That shot of encouragement always helped me press on. Even though I never met many of these encouraging people face to face, they were true mentors to me. I want to pass on the good gifts they gave me by helping others understand the power and significance of caring labors.

I would like to invite you into my own journey of discovering that caring for others is real work and real art. Caregiving is a creative, God-given approach to life. It is love in the midst of life's extraordinary dailiness, the creation of beauty in the rhythm of our unique relationships. We were created to have caregiving lives.

My hope is that reading this book will broaden and affirm your understanding of caregiving in all its diversity. We cannot separate real demonstrations of care from the gospel itself. When we care for people in imaginative, life-giving ways, we embody the love of Jesus. What could be a grander calling?

ONE

A MISUNDERSTOOD ART

What Does It Mean to Give Care?

Every person is an artist. The whole of life is a creative act. The warp and woof of each life is equivalent to the artist's paint or the musician's sounds.

—RANALD MACAULAY and JERRAM BARRS, *Being Human*

When I married my high-school sweetheart in 1975, I was completely unprepared for the stream of people needing care that would come my way in the years ahead. The furthest thing from my mind as a nineteen-year-old bride was any thought or understanding of the labor, expertise, and artistry that would emerge as I responded to those needs. It would take years before I realized that making a home and caring for a husband and children was real work—work that was physical, intellectual, spiritual, and creative. Time would add the challenge and responsibility of caring for other people in myriad ways: in the frequent practice of hospitality, as an employer, a neighbor, a daughter with a dying mother, a friend, a volunteer in the community, a church member.

The philosophy and skill I would need to carry out this calling was not something I had considered while taking vocational tests in high school.

My experience as a young person was similar to the experiences of many others. I learned a few skills but had no broad overview of caregiving and why it mattered. As a young woman I had the tools for thinking about the possibilities of paid work in the marketplace, but I didn't know how to prepare for or value unpaid caretaking responsibilities. It took years for me to realize that the many faces of caregiving would be a central part of my life's work.

"JUST" A CAREGIVER?

Caregiving is part of most people's lives on some level. God appointed us to a caregiving lifestyle when he created us to love and to desire relationship. When we love others, we want to provide for them, to show our love by caring for them as individuals. Caregiving touches many aspects of life—everything from the creation of a meal, to how we care for each other in sickness and old age, to the importance we give to celebrations and hospitality, to the way we live as a friend and neighbor.

For many people caregiving is full-time work. Full-time caregiving in its many forms can be difficult to describe in the usual introductory conversations when people ask the question, "What do you do?" Most caregivers are at a loss to know how to answer. We know we're exhausted at the end of a day, but knowing how to explain the exact nature of our work is baffling. The work is varied, and each new day or season brings with it a different set of needs.

The imagination and labor required of a mother who's learning to soothe and care for her first baby is quite different from that of an adult son who's caring for his increasingly dependent father. Both caregivers are learning that the work is physically demanding, intellectually challenging, and engages the imagination, but describing it is difficult. Much of this labor is invisible to others, and because of this, it's often left out of conversations about work, calling, and individual contributions to the common good of society.

Our culture sends a strong message that success equals the attainment of wealth or recognition, whether in business or ministry. This idea is so deeply ingrained in our thinking that people who are quietly and faithfully caring for one life at a time behind the scenes wonder if anyone considers the work of their hands and heart to be of value. A young mother I know who recently changed the focus of her work from the marketplace to the care of her home, husband, and their first child, said to me in reference to her caregiving, "I don't even know if it matters to God." The fact that she would even have to wonder about this is a terrible consequence of the distorted thinking that has taken root over the generations.

Mothers coming from other careers to do the full-time work of family caregiving often speak of an identity crisis stemming from dismissive cultural attitudes. But this crisis extends to anyone in a caregiving vocation, especially one that is difficult to name.

Last summer I met a woman at a retreat in Texas. As we were exchanging pleasantries while waiting in the food line, I asked about her life. She seemed almost apologetic that she didn't have a title that would easily identify her work. She told me that she spent most of her time taking care of her husband. He had an illness requiring her full-time attention. I knew by the way she tiptoed into the subject that she thought I wouldn't understand that this could be the work of her days.

This woman was probably used to questions and comments like the one I received while accompanying my husband to a speaking engagement at a university. I was conversing with one of the students—a young woman—when she said to me: "Do you *do* anything or are you *just* a housewife?" Frankly, I was floored by her words and the ignorance they revealed, particularly when she told me that her own mother was a homemaker. Christian teaching was the foundation of this university, yet this young woman had failed to make the intellectual connection that service to Jesus takes place in all of life and certainly does not exclude the realm of the home.

Even our language reflects society's warped view of caregiving. For instance, we refer to a person who does not work for pay outside the home as "nonworking." This is rarely an accurate description of someone, and it steals dignity from a person made in God's image as a worker. The word "housewife" comes up short as well. After all, what woman was ever married to her house? Even the terms "stay-at-home mom" and "stay-at-home dad" are inaccurate titles. They are widely used today to differentiate between parents who leave home to do paid work and parents who work from home, either with no pay or because they are self-employed. "Stay-at-home mom" and "stay-at-home dad" are passive sounding titles for people whose work is filled with purpose and activity. Parents in this position are based at home, but they come and go frequently in the course of a busy week. They are also a huge source of volunteer help for schools, churches, and communities, which takes them away from home. We have forgotten that leaving home for the day and earning a salary are not the only indications that someone is a worker.

A large portion of the population is left with the feeling that their work has no value. David Westcott underscores this problem in his book *Work Well, Live Well.* He suggests that women who introduce themselves as "only a housewife" illustrate his point. As Westcott writes, these are "extremely capable women who do an incredibly important job yet apologize for their existence."[1]

Before I had the language to talk about my vocation, I would often feel left out of the conversation when the topic of work came up in a group. *I* knew how hard I was working, but most of the people I met identified work as something you went away from home to do and got paid for. My caring work took place in many settings, but I wasn't paid to do it, so in the eyes of those in my own culture, I was not a legitimate worker.

As I saw the distorted picture society, as a whole, had of caregiving and how my own caregiving gifts and activities were devalued, it became increasingly clear to me that the art of caregiving is becoming a casualty of this dismissive attitude.

The Price of Progress

We were created to respond to voice, touch, and physical presence, yet our society is increasingly voiceless, faceless, and untouchable. We can bank, shop, put gas in the car, buy groceries, and make business calls without once interacting with a live person. Most of the time it's convenient, many times it's frustrating, but all of it contributes to the loss of human connection in daily life.

Societal structures are efficient but not always beneficial to the emotional and physical health of the people they are meant to serve. Technological advances bring help, physical healing, and convenience, but they also invade our daily routines and patterns. High-tech industries subtly change the way we think and act until we have fewer and fewer opportunities for face-to-face human connection. Mounting time pressures make it easier for us to be isolated and unaware of each other's needs, resulting in a thread of loneliness and neglect that runs through our lives.

As the gap widens between family and community needs and the people who are available to meet those needs, we are left scrambling for substitutes. We've entered the era of home meal replacements, domestic outsourcing, and outside care for our elders and children. We are growing accustomed to writing a check for services that have historically been done out of love. We are in danger of losing a vision for the creative, interdisciplinary, hands-on work of loving each other deeply.

We sometimes seem to have forgotten that though society is constantly shifting and adapting to new ways, it will always be filled with human beings who need personal care and attention. We should carefully consider the difference between service that is motivated by love and concern for the individual, and service that is purchased from anonymous, for-profit companies. Important issues are at stake. When we give care personally, out of love, we are affirming two key truths:

1. *Human needs are complex.* We are physical, intellectual, psychological, and spiritual beings. Caregivers use the diverse body of knowledge and skill they've acquired and design their work around the needs of the whole person or family. A business, on the other hand, must specialize, usually in only one kind of service. Without access to a range of services or the means to pay for them, human need falls through the cracks.

2. *The flesh and bones of what it means to love is passed down through generations of people, not businesses.* In 1 Timothy 5:3-16, Paul instructs his readers to provide for their immediate and extended families. This encompasses more than financial provision. Paul is referring to a holistic care, which is a mixture of monetary support and personal attention. Human beings need both. To *provide* means to see needs in advance, to think broadly and work for the benefit of loved ones on many different levels. The basic human hungers for continuity, comfort, connection, security, and beauty are also needs and are met through the details of caregiving.

When we recognize that the work of caregiving is essential to human well-being, we take the first step toward easing the loneliness and neglect that characterizes so many lives today. One writer reminds us,

We do not have to go back many generations to remember that "women's work" was not merely labor spent doing things inside the house but also the role of creating and sustaining the bonds of affection and support in the whole community. If this work is being done poorly today—as most observers will agree it is despite massive government expenditures—a renewed appreciation for it *as work* and therefore as conferring adult power, dignity, and responsibility would restore to women (and perhaps also some men) the incentive to play this role. If work were separated from pay but not from honor, people whose necessities were provided in some other way would not be ashamed to work for free.[2]

It's ironic that the very thing society is groaning for is what caregivers have to offer—yet we're more apt to hear of the need for more government programs than to hear support and encouragement for caregivers.

Caring work is a vital service to humanity; it is never trivial or disposable. Imagine what life would be like without the caregiving that is given freely in so many different ways. I know a retired man who spends large chunks of each day taking care of his elderly neighbors. He checks in on many of them daily, visiting those who are lonely, making repairs in their homes, and seeing that they get to their doctor's appointments. These people know they have someone to call on when they're in need. What would this neighborhood be like without this man's care? Though it may seem like caregivers are fading from the landscape, in truth there are people everywhere who are engaged in the art and work of caring.

GIVING CARE

I've come to understand that an essential step toward recognizing and encouraging caregivers—on an individual as well as a corporate level—is to understand what caregiving means and why we are drawn to give care.

The work of giving care takes different shapes and forms in individual lives. While caregiving is often associated with women, it's clear from the Scriptures that all God's children are responsible to take neighbor-love out

nd bring it into our concrete, daily lives. Our overarching
kingdom of God is to take care of the earth and its people,
to protect and develop what God has made. Within this broad directive is
the distinctive calling to care for families, neighbors, friends, and communities. In the parable of the good Samaritan (Luke 10:25-37), the real
neighbor was the traveler who provided just what the injured man on the
road needed—bandages, medicine, transportation, and money to pay his
expenses for further care. It was holistic and embodied care.

As caregivers to the world—those in whom the love of Christ and the
love of people are intertwined—we are called to remain alert to the fabric
of human design. Every person created in the image of God longs to be
cared for in tangible ways, whether they realize it or not. With kindness
and consideration becoming less common, we need to preserve these
timeless manifestations of simple care. We can do this by cultivating an
increased sensitivity to the gentle power of the personal touch. We can take
the initiative to look strangers in the eye and speak a greeting. We can initiate conversation in the checkout line at the grocery store. It takes effort
to treat fellow human beings with dignity, especially if they don't return it,
but this is what it means to give care?

Dreaming, praying, and working for—in a sense, *imagining* for—a
good story in the lives of those whose paths we cross briefly or for the
long haul is what we're made for. Paul wrote to the church in Galatia,
"as we have opportunity, let us do good to all people" (Galatians 6:10;
see also 1 Corinthians 10:24). We are "created in Christ Jesus to do good
works" (Ephesians 2:10). Sometimes the good we can do is simply to treat
a stranger with kindness. And for those we walk with over the course of
a lifetime, the possibilities for contributing to one another's lives are endless. We are meant to add to the lives of others. Everything we do, from
pursuing the difficult, messy work of forgiveness and reconciliation to
imagining and creating a party, is important and worthwhile.

In *The Mark of the Christian,* Francis Schaeffer writes about the connection of the gospel to real, everyday demonstrations of love. In his words, "The observable practice of truth and the observable practice of love go hand in hand with the proclamation of the good news of Jesus Christ."[3] Friends or coworkers will know they're loved when you take the time to bake their birthday cake, deliver food to them when they're ill, or listen quietly when they're in pain. As Christian people, we know the worth of the individual. We know what it means to serve Jesus by serving others in very personal ways. We are commanded to love, and love takes place in real life, where concrete choices and actions show people they matter.

A GOD OF BEAUTY

Though our individual gifts differ, our desire to care, our ability to care, and our need to care exist because of one common truth: Our God is a caring God. We care because we were made in his image.

One of the ways God's image is reflected in us is through our need for beauty. We were created to love the beautiful. Beauty gives pleasure to the senses, lifts the mind and spirit, and brings us to a place of longing for the Creator of all beauty.

Caring often means bringing beautiful things into people's lives—cutting flowers for them, cleaning their house, taking them to see the ocean. Our desire for beauty is a reflection of a God who loves the beautiful. God has set us down in a crazy, amazing world full of breathtaking sights and sounds and scents and textures, most of which seem to exist only for his pleasure and ours. When beauty is offered as a gift of love, what is seen or heard or tasted goes past the surface and into the heart.

But with such a high value placed on speed and getting things done in the quickest way possible, the creation of beauty is not "practical" in our culture today. Consider strip malls. The buildings are inexpensive and easy to put up, but they add nothing to the aesthetics or inspiration of a community. Commenting on the spirit of pragmatism in our Western society, Dr. Leland Ryken notes, "Cities followed the course of what was efficient and useful, not what was beautiful and enjoyable and humanly enriching."[4] The movement of our culture toward the ugly and even the grotesque can be seen and heard in music, film, and fashion, in ways we treat the body, and in attitudes and ideas about our humanity. In a multitude of ways, through cheap imitations and settling for substitutes, we become divorced from the way we're made.

In small and large ways, when we create beauty—in our environment, relationships, music, cooking, poetry, and celebrations—we push back the effects of the Fall and express our hope for the new heaven and new earth that God promises. When we give artful attention to detail, we point people to a truer and better reality. When we offer beauty, we touch something in the human soul. We remind others of who they are and what they were made for. We bring hope and inspiration. This is a way of caring.

A part of reflecting God's beauty is recognizing and celebrating the beauty of his character. We serve a God of creativity, sacrifice, and extravagance. We, too, are called to reflect these characteristics as we live out the truth of what it means to give care.

A Creative God

I lived for years around artistic types—musicians, painters, photographers—without ever realizing that I myself had creative abilities. I wasn't an artist in the classic sense; I couldn't paint a picture to save my life. But when our children were very young, somewhere around four and seven years old, I read a book by Edith Schaeffer titled *Hidden Art*.[5] It is a unique and inspirational book that points out the many opportunities for creativity and artistic expression in the ordinary places of daily life. Since we have been made in the image of God, the Creator of all the diversity and beauty in the universe, part of our image-bearing capacity is to create. We have an inner urge to do so. It was as I read *Hidden Art* that I realized I was made in the image of the Supreme Artist and *could* make all sorts of artful choices about how to live and how to care for others.

Recognizing that God calls me to be creative because *he* is creative stirred my imagination and cultivated my creativity. Caring work is a creative and artistic expression of who we are in Christ. God calls us to care imaginatively, to ask, How can I go the extra mile in this situation? How can I more creatively love this person? How can I reflect my own artistic individuality in how I relate and act?

The choices can be very simple ones—homemade chocolate cake instead of a packaged mix, cut greenery from the yard for the table, a mass of twinkling votive candles in the living room. A little imagination, for example, transforms a meal from basic care of the body into a memorable experience. To quote a good friend, the meal becomes first aid to the soul.

We can also be creative in hundreds of ways in our caregiving away from home. We can assist someone in a move by packing, lugging boxes, or dropping in at lunchtime with a bag of hamburgers and fries. We can drive a coworker to get his car fixed or tutor kids after school. My daughter works for a public television station that is located next to a grammar school. She and some of her coworkers take off half an hour from work two days a week to read books to the younger students. These activities may seem mundane in some ways, but actually, they are opportunities for us to respond to God's call to creativity as he draws us to be more like him.

A Sacrificial God

In the book of Matthew we read about a woman who poured a jar of very expensive perfume on Jesus' head. When the disciples saw this, they asked, "Why this waste?" (26:8). Jesus replied, "Why are you bothering this woman? She has done a beautiful thing to me" (verse 10). This woman loved Jesus by giving him something extremely valuable—giving not just in drops or moments with something left over for herself, but completely, all at once. She cared for him not just in the giving of perfume but in the fact that she was losing something by giving. She wanted to honor who he was by making a personal sacrifice. In loving sacrificially, she reflected God's sacrificial love—the same love God showed when he sent his own Son to die for us on the cross.

We may not be called to pour perfume over someone's head, but we are often called to offer something far more valuable in today's culture: time. Sometimes we—or others—may see the giving of our time as a waste. Shouldn't we be spending our time, energy, and money on something with a more tangible result? Caring for people involves the sacrifice of time. It means taking opportunities to demonstrate love because an opportunity may not come again. We have a finite number of minutes and hours in our earthly life, but we can do things that count for all eternity.

An Extravagant God

The film *Babette's Feast* is the story of a French chef who experiences an unexpected financial windfall and uses all her earnings to create an elaborate, multicourse feast for a group of poor villagers. The villagers were caught inside a lawgiving, burdensome religious system, and the meal was unlike anything they have ever experienced. They were reserved and shocked at first, but eventually they melted into Babette's extreme expression of love, grace, and gratitude for them. The days of work, the talent, the money, the artistry, all that was poured out on their behalf was a truer picture of God's love than any the villagers have ever known.

God our Father offers love without reserve to his children. "How great is the love the Father has lavished on us, that we should be called children of God!" (1 John 3:1). He shows his love for us through his abundant mercy and unending grace.

We, too, can reflect God's extravagant love, even when the things we do for others seem small. Stopping to listen to someone when you're in a hurry, helping a neighbor unload groceries from the car, sending roses to a friend when a card would do—each act is a generous expression of care. Other times the lavish caring comes with planning and forethought. You want to do something that communicates to people that you've thought of them in advance. When there's an occasion to celebrate—an anniversary, a graduation, a retirement—you take the extra time, plan for weeks, cook the favorite meal and desserts, go all out in the decorating. It's a lot of work, but your extravagance in caring says, "This is my opportunity to show you through my efforts and my artistry how much I love you. Because I love you so much, I will not hold back; I will give my all."

FILLING THE GAP

Our culture places a lot of emphasis on image—the way we look, the clothes we wear, the cars we drive. In short, we are most concerned with how we present ourselves to the world. When we give more attention to image than to content, depth, or quality of heart and mind, we don't easily understand the idea of bringing forth beauty from the inside of a person or in human relationships.

My friend Nita Andrews—a family counselor, public speaker, and wife and mother—offers these wise words: "If we go towards individualism, our biographies will be boring. We'll be degraded along with our gifts and talents." On the other hand, if we reach toward people, we're ushered into a way of life that has unlimited creative potential and no room for waste and boredom. Seeking the good of another person fills our lives with purpose and meaning.

Whether we are engaged in the vocation of caregiving or are recipients of someone's caregiving gifts and talents, we need to understand and respect the vital role this kind of work plays in our society. We need to legitimize unpaid caregiving vocations, encouraging those who are called to fill the important roles that God has assigned.

As our society grows increasingly technological, consumer-oriented, isolated, and lonely, those who take their caregiving gifts and callings seriously can fill a tremendous void. If you are someone whose primary work is to care physically and emotionally for those entrusted to you, then you are in the business of imagining for the good of those people and working to bring about what is true and lovely and admirable in them. Your gifts, your time, and your work are important. You are not alone. Like countless others throughout generations, you are participating in God's perfect design to love in the everyday realities of life. In doing so you reflect the beauty of a God whose love knows no limit.

TWO

✠✠✠✠✠✠✠✠

GOD'S GRAND ADVENTURE

Caring Is a Calling

> Could mere loving be a life's work? Could it be a career like marriage or nursing the sick or going on the stage? Could it be an adventure?
>
> —ELIZABETH GOUDGE's character Mary in *The Dean's Watch*

Even after I realized how many people in my life would need care, it took years before I understood that the word "calling" could apply to me. The word was thrown around rather haphazardly and seemed to land on people with careers in the arts, music, medicine, or the pastorate, but it didn't come anywhere near someone like me. What I did was hard to name and hard to explain. When I tried to name it myself, the most accurate description I could come up with was "caring work." I take care of people. I'm a caregiver.

In 1996 I set out to understand the subject of work and calling, to see what it meant for me and for others whose lives had a similar bent. Prior to that time, my work doing home-based accounting and administration for our family music business had grown into a full-time position. Though I had always worked in various ways for our business—and still do—when the work became full time, I grew increasingly frustrated and

19

discontent, and often bitter and resentful. The reason: I was spending my days working in an area I was not drawn to, not gifted for, and would never have chosen had it not been connected to my husband and our family income. I was just filling a need that kept getting bigger and bigger. Neither my husband nor I stopped to consider whether I was the right person for the job. As time went on, I realized with deepening clarity that the music business was my husband's calling, but it wasn't mine, apart from the larger view of coming alongside him as his life partner.

When I reached a crisis point, I learned of a class that psychologist Dr. Bruce McCurdy was leading. The class topic was "Life Purpose and Life Planning." For the first time I began to look at my personality type, my gifts, the settings I preferred to work in, the tools I like to use, fields of knowledge I already had, and others I would like to pursue. I thought about the things I love to do and will always do in some capacity because they are integral to who I am. I began to understand that those things are inside me because God has put them there. I would be wise to pay attention.

ANSWERING THE CALL

Three areas of calling stood out to me as I worked through the class material: writing, gardening, and caregiving. Within a short time, I knew that I should purposefully move toward each one.

When the timing was right, we hired someone to take over my work in our company. I had no crystal clear vision of where I was headed, but I started by taking steps in each area. My caregiving role was already in place, but my efforts had been frustrated by time constraints. Now without the full days of office work, I was freed up to give myself more intentionally to caregiving—in our home and family, with our friends, and later through the women's ministry in my church. I also took classes through the University of Tennessee Agricultural Extension Service and became a

Master Gardener. And I began researching and writing this book. I had no idea at the time that I would ever have the privilege of publishing it. I just knew I was strongly compelled to make sense out of this topic that was so huge in my life and in the lives of many others I knew and observed.

In my research I read books by Os Guinness, Paul Marshall, Leland Ryken, Lee Hardy, and Elton Trueblood. I listened to audio lectures by Dick and Mardi Keyes from L'Abri Fellowship, and Dan Doriani and Esther Meek from Covenant Theological Seminary. The scholarship of these teachers helped me understand my life and settle into it with greater purpose.

I found that *calling* and *vocation* mean the same thing—one comes from a Latin root and the other from an Anglo-Saxon root. According to Lee Hardy, in the New Testament,

> the primary, if not exclusive, meaning of the term "vocation"—or calling *(klēsis)*—pertains to the call of the gospel, pure and simple.... Here we are not being asked to choose from a variety of callings, to decide which one is "right" for us. Rather one call goes out to all— the call of discipleship. For it is incumbent upon all Christians to follow Christ, and, in so doing, to become the kind of people God wants us to be.

Hardy goes on to write that, as Christians, we are "commanded, and therefore called, to love and serve our neighbors with the gifts that God has given us."[1]

Martin Luther and John Calvin made enormous contributions to the concept of *vocation*. Luther wrote that our vocations come to us through the stations of life in which God has placed us, and through which we love our neighbor as ourselves. Our stations may or may not include paid occupations but do include the many ways we relate to others—as a husband or wife, a child, a parent, a church member, a citizen. Calvin added to this concept by saying that God has given each person specific gifts and talents that should be used for the sake of others.

Calling does not refer to just one job or one task. It encompasses the whole shape of our life: the web of relationships and diversity of work that God gives to each Christian. The Christian's primary calling is to follow Christ. We are called first to him. Subordinate to and connected with our first calling come our secondary callings, such as homemaking, dentistry, parenting, filmmaking, farming, or politics.

Different aspects of our callings unfold over a lifetime. I love Os Guinness's succinct definition: "Calling is the truth that God calls us to himself so decisively that everything we are, everything we do, and everything we have is invested with a special devotion and dynamism lived out as a response to his summons and service."[2] Calling is a comprehensive picture of the unique path laid out for each of us, consisting of the particular things God has asked us—and sometimes no one else—to do.

PATTERNS OF CALLING

Since the path laid out before us is uniquely ours, we must pay attention to what God is showing us through our relationships, our inclinations, our natural and spiritual gifts, and life circumstances. What is the story of our life telling us?

Looking back over the last twenty years of my life, I see that my calling to care weaves in and out of my other callings. It's clear to me now that caregiving is part of my makeup. It's the way God has made me to respond to the world.

Whether we consider caregiving as a lifestyle or a distinct vocation, the call to care encompasses three broad categories.

1. *Regardless of vocation, everyone who follows Christ is called to
   live in such a way that love is embodied and real to other people.*

We are called to a lifestyle of caring. We have an overarching purpose that informs everything we do: We are caregivers and truth tellers to the world. Our love of Christ and love of people are intertwined and lived out in hundreds of specific, creative ways over a lifetime. Caring flows from being attuned to the personal needs of individuals. No matter what kind of work occupies the main part of our day, no matter what our gifts and talents are, we can approach the people around us with an attitude of care. When caregiving doesn't come naturally, it's not a time for self-condemnation but for learning, for leaning on God in the challenge, for not shirking responsibility but finding ways to give care that are congruent with our gifts and abilities.

2. *In some relationships, caregiving is intensive only for a period of time.* Though we are always called to care, sometimes our calling is more specific and clear for a limited amount of time. Parenting, for example, requires a concentrated focus of eighteen or nineteen years for each child. Once children are grown and out of the house, the call to give care is still there, but the time requirements are much different. Likewise, an adult child with elderly parents or other relatives in need is a caregiver for a specific period of time. The caregiving is temporary, not lifelong. A friend walking closely with another friend through a life-threatening illness provides support and care only for a season.

3. *Sometimes caregiving is a vocation—a lifework—that manifests itself over a lifetime.* Skill and talent coupled with a built-in longing to respond to human need with practical, creative service, produces a caregiving vocation. This may result when expertise develops unexpectedly through caring for someone during an intense period of time or when an individual

simply has a God-given set of gifts and talents. Some of God's people have specific caregiving gifts: They relate and listen well. They are gifted at creating beautiful and nurturing environments. They are drawn to care for the sick or dying. They have spiritual gifts of helps, mercy, and encouragement. They are excellent cooks, generous in practicing hospitality, or continually use their creativity to serve others in a multitude of ways. Those who are called to give care and pursue it intentionally bear much fruit in their lives that they may or may not be privileged to see.

In Os Guinness's words, "As we make our contribution along the line of our gifts and callings, and others do the same, there is both a fruitfulness and a rest in the outcome. Our gifts are used for the purpose for which they were given us. And we can rest in doing what we can without ever pretending we are more than the little people we plainly are."[3] The question each of us must ask is, Are we faithful to our callings? The rest is up to God.

A CAREGIVING JOURNEY

Woven throughout our lives are these overarching and specific callings to care. As our relationship with Jesus deepens, we often hear more clearly our call to love others through action. Seasons of more intensive caregiving are sometimes planned but are often unexpected. If we are particularly gifted in caring for others, we may be aware of that gifting in childhood, or we may discover it well into adulthood.

During different times in my life caregiving has taken different forms, but over the years I've realized that my personal call is to a caring *vocation*—caregiving is my lifework. I understand it now as a calling, but the clarity was slow in coming. When I married my husband, Chuck (many of you may know him as recording artist and producer Charlie Peacock), I had only a vague concept of what it meant to care for him or anyone else. I made lavish promises to love, honor, and cherish him, but I had no resources to carry out my vows.

For the first seven years of our marriage, Chuck and I patched together a philosophy of life, borrowing ideas from radical feminism, a mix of Eastern religions, and our favorite novelists and poets. The core ideas from the women's movement helped me understand that my life was full of dignity and possibility. But as I grew more radical and extreme in my thinking, I came to believe that my rights were at the center of the universe.

In the beginning Chuck and I were idealistic about a future that would bring us into an intimate union while keeping our individual identities and rights intact. However, as the years added up, the consequences of putting self at the center of a relationship that demands just the opposite were disastrous.

The recreational drinking and drugs we indulged in led to addiction, financial ruin, and marital breakdown. We moved from job to job, school to school, baby-sitter to baby-sitter, and house to house, never committing to anyone or anything past its ability to keep us interested. We gave no attention to the details of family life. We painted in broad strokes and did just enough to get by—tending to the most basic needs of food and clean clothes, but not much more. Living without a larger story to guide us, we floundered without intent and purpose.

Our entrance into the Christian life in the seventh year of our marriage was the beginning of a profound change that affected everything about how we thought, worked, created, and loved. The spiritual awakening that began in a program of recovery and culminated with our conversion to Christianity awakened parts of me that had lain dormant.

Though I didn't set out to become a homemaker and, in fact, in my past had a dismissive attitude toward women with that title, I slowly realized that this work was important and necessary to the health of our family. We were coming out of a chaotic life, the result of our first seven years of marriage. As the image of God in me was stirred, I wanted to shape beauty and order from our chaos.

A new appreciation for the intricacies of nurturing accompanied and stimulated my intellectual curiosity. Raising a family took on new meaning, and the days seemed full of possibility. Chuck and I opened our eyes to the need for breadwinning *and* caregiving. We divided our labor according to the particularities of our life and viewed each area with fresh respect.

With a clear mind and a new sense of purpose, Chuck was taking every opportunity to earn money and repair the state of our finances. As a musician, this meant that he was often gone at night and on weekends, in the studio or traveling for gigs. So I learned to take care of the bookkeeping and paperwork generated by his self-employment. As I also learned to run a household and care for two small children, I found myself working harder than I ever had before.

Our children, Molly and Sam, were nearly two and five years old and had never known the safety net of a nurturing home. We had lived haphazardly, never putting forth any effort to create a living space that would nurture, inspire, and enable us to care well for each other. Our previous motto had been taken from the feminist bumper sticker we had on our car: "The Revolution Begins at Home." Seeking to break down sexual stereotypes on the home front, Chuck and I had mentally kept score of whether our partner had done his or her fair share of household work. When there was failure on either side, no grace or help was given—the work was simply left undone.

If, for example, it was Chuck's turn to do the dishes and he hadn't done them, I would wait him out. When I was hungry I washed a plate, fork, and glass—just enough dishes for *my* meal—and left the rest. When enough days and dishes stacked up, we could not enter the kitchen for the stench. Usually after an argument, one or both of us would begrudgingly cave in and deal with the mess. This diseased way of living had spread itself over the whole of our home life, and the places we lived in reflected the overall confusion of our life.

Life in Christ was like breathing new air. Our household came alive. Chuck and I were working together for the preservation of our family, and individual rights could no longer be the driving force behind our choices. Danielle Crittenden puts it well:

> The two adults suddenly find themselves at the helm of a new unit, a new team, whose success will depend upon their wholehearted commitment to each other and to their children. Whether the new arrangement is strictly "fair" to any individual within it ceases to be important, or becomes less important than whether it is "best" or "right" for the family as a whole.[4]

We were gaining an understanding that sacrificial work was required from both of us in order to serve a larger purpose.

Family Needs

In my new work of homemaking, I found myself responding with an eager mind and willing hands. A button of creativity was pushed inside me as I started imagining ways to nurture my family. I was learning the importance of caring for their immediate needs while simultaneously creating memories that would carry over into their future.

Motherhood became an adventure in guiding my children and watching their gifts and personalities emerge. G. K. Chesterton's book *What's Wrong with the World?* speaks to the awful misconception that being home with young children is drudgery. Putting the task in proper perspective, Chesterton points out that women (and I would add men) who are surrounded by very young children are with those "who require to be taught not so much anything as everything. Babies need not to be taught a trade, but to be introduced to the world." He continues:

> When domesticity, for instance, is called drudgery, all the difficulty arises from a double meaning in the word. If drudgery only means dreadfully hard work, I admit the woman drudges in the home, as a man might drudge at the Cathedral of Amiens or drudge behind a gun at Trafalgar. But if it means that the hard work is more heavy because it is trifling, colorless and of small import to the soul,...
> I give it up; I do not know what the words mean. To be Queen Elizabeth within a definite area, deciding sales, banquets, labors and holidays; to be Whitely within a certain area, providing toys, boots, sheets, cakes, and books; to be Aristotle within a certain area, teaching morals, manners, theology, and hygiene; I can understand how this might exhaust the mind, but I cannot imagine how it could narrow it.[5]

Chesterton goes on to ask, "How can it be a large career to tell other people's children about the Rule of Three, and a small career to tell one's own children about the universe?"[6]

My own thoughts echoed Chesterton's as I began to imagine teaching my own children about a subject matter as huge as the whole universe. The seeds of a new philosophy that were planted in those early years of our Christian life would bud and flower with time. All the seemingly unrelated tasks I was learning, such as cooking, paying the bills on time, creating art projects and games for the children, taking them on field trips, providing clean clothes and a clean house for my family, planting flowers, reading bedtime stories, and planning picnics and holidays, were not unrelated at all. When woven together over time, they would create a strong undergirding, a tapestry of color, delicious tastes and smells, belly laughter, trust, security, order, beauty, and connection.

Growing Relationships

Our home quickly became a place where caring for the needs of more people than just our little family was necessary. God brought people into our life who needed a place to stay for a night, a week, a month. I learned that hospitality was a holistic endeavor that included feeding people, cleaning up after them, and being available as a listener late into the night yet still getting up in the morning to care for the children. While it could be exhausting work, I found satisfaction and joy in being involved with people and with the deepening of our relationships.

My call to caring work grew in diversity as we got involved with a church body. The Christian believers who first embraced our family were a warm group of people who cared for each other's needs in many ways. Whenever there was a family with a new baby, a home where someone was sick or hospitalized, or a family grieving the loss of a loved one, the women, in particular, in that church were quick to organize meals, housecleaning help, or baby-sitting.

Under the tutelage of these women, I learned to care for the practical needs of the body of Christ. When cooking and delivering meals, I learned to consider the needs of the people I was serving. I planned a fairly simple meal for a family with five children and offered more adventuresome food to a single person or a couple who would enjoy a different kind of treat. I tried new recipes and learned to think about combinations of flavors and colors when presenting a meal meant to nourish body and soul. Artful attention to detail would refresh people in a greater way than simply meeting their basic needs for food.

My caring work extended into the community, where I volunteered in my children's schools. Being involved in the schools was a natural extension of caring for my own children and staying in touch with their life away from home, as well as a way of offering care to other people's children.

I also found ways to respond to something God had placed in me as a little girl. When I was very young, I accompanied one of my stepsisters to her job as a nurse's aide in a convalescent hospital. I spent my time there visiting with the patients and struck up a friendship with one of them, maintaining it through correspondence when I went back to my home state. From that point on I was drawn to older people and loved spending time with them. I volunteered in a hospital during high school and worked in nursing homes before and after my marriage. After Chuck and I became Christians, I had a growing desire to ease the loneliness of others and realized we had a nursing home close to our house. I began volunteering there, spending time with people who rarely or never had visitors. The kids often accompanied me, and seeds of compassion were planted in them that continue to flower in their adult lives.

For years after that experience, I continued to be a visitor in nursing homes. One year, through a serendipitous phone call, I started taking groceries to an older woman who was housebound. As long as she had someone to bring her groceries, she could continue to live on her own. I would add her grocery list to mine and then stay for conversation when I made the delivery.

Later years would bring me new opportunities and new ways to respond to God's call. Sometimes I gave care in my neighborhood; at other times I focused more on my church, my friendships, or my extended family. God strengthened my caregiving gifts and desires as he opened my eyes to the needs of others. Looking back I see his grace gently guiding me to a fuller understanding of his call to give care.

A DIVERSITY OF GIFTS

These are my roots, the beginnings of a caregiving life with different manifestations for different seasons. My call to caring is different from that of other people because our callings are so varied. As God's representatives, we have thousands of places and ways to shine. To serve God effectively, we must be led individually by the Spirit.

Linda is a high-school teacher from my hometown who has a life calling to care for her community. In partnership with her husband, Bud, she's been patching the holes of need for people in her town for years. Her care is practical and creative. It has ranged from taking in students who needed a home to delivering freshly baked bread on a weekly basis to an invalid who needed to experience the love of God. Linda's stories could fill a whole book, but I'll select just a few and let her describe in her own words a few of her caring encounters, reflecting her unique call. Linda tells me,

> One neat opportunity to care came when a prostitute and her pimp who found Jesus decided to get married. I had no part in leading them to him but did get involved (on one day's notice) with the wedding. We stripped people's gardens and managed to put together a quiet but sweet little wedding at the church. Just after the marriage, she was diagnosed with TB, and I did a Bible study with her in the hospital. I had to put on a sterile gown, mask, and booties to go in with her. It was a blessed time for me. I felt very privileged to watch the Lord "clean up" this young woman.
>
> I also had a chance to participate in God's care for a woman who was diagnosed with ovarian cancer and had to have surgery and chemo. She was a member of our church, but I didn't know her. I called and told her that I would be her "food fairy" while she was doing chemo and would cook anything that she had a craving for. It took some convincing that I actually meant it, but we really had fun and became friends as well. I got requests for some strange things: three-layer chocolate cake and guacamole. Chemo so often takes the taste buds and the appetite, so getting people to eat is really important.

Linda also tells of how Bud loves to make soup of all kinds. "In the winter especially, he hauls out the soup pots on Saturdays or on Sundays after church and makes gallons! We take the soup to people who are sick or depressed or alone or who just need a special touch."

Given the self-centered world we're immersed in, Linda's story is unusual. I asked about her philosophy. What had driven her to create the space and time necessary to respond to such diverse needs? She answered,

> How could I not? I was so grateful when Jesus came into my life in such a magnificent way. I just asked to be used. I believe that he uses us according to our personalities and gifts. I'm an extrovert who finds it easy to talk to people. I'm intuitive to people's needs and have a desire to help them become all they can be. To me, the joy lies in the journey and in the obedience. Bud and I both have gifts of hospitality and service. It just comes naturally. People call and tell us about someone, and we go, or they just appear.

Linda's comments are a great help in understanding individual caregiving vocations. Her gifts, outgoing personality, and like-minded marriage partner make her willing and able to do things that others couldn't. Her reliance on God's direction keeps her from straining to go where he hasn't called her.

Linda also has wise words about the motivation behind our caregiving acts: "One thing's for sure: Don't do it if the Holy Spirit isn't directing you. If it's done in the flesh, it's awful. If it's done for approval, it's awful. It becomes a burden, and no one gets blessed. It's worse than not doing anything." This is so important to remember. It is the essence of calling. God calls us individually, and we're accountable to him alone. He calls us to act out of obedience to him, motivated not by obligation or a desire for power and recognition, but because we want to bring glory to him by loving others.

I love the fact that God uses our unique personalities and giftings, the geographical places we live, and the needs of our particular families and communities to direct our caregiving. I can rest in who I am and be inspired by a story like Linda's, but I don't need to try to replicate what she does. I can trust God to bring to me those who need my particular brand of care rather than falling under a burden of guilt by comparing my calling to someone else's.

My friend Kathi's caregiving path includes her work as a wife and mother, the caring she does as a gifted chef, and the role she has played as a "patient advocate," helping a number of family members and friends through serious illness and death. "Not everyone is a natural caregiver," Kathi offers. "When confronted with caregiving for sick people, ask yourself, 'Am I the right person for this task?' There are many different levels of care to participate in. Some people make better 'backup' caregivers. These roles are just as valid and give the primary person time away for rejuvenation."

Another friend whose gifts are very different from Linda's or Kathi's explained to me, "I'm not a high-energy go-getter, but I'm learning that I can care for people through quietness and that I feel cared for through other people's quietness as well." Each contribution of care is necessary and significant to the huge story of redemption that God is telling in human history.

CELEBRATING THE GIFT

God gives us the great gift of joy in doing what we are called to do. Sometimes we recognize our callings most clearly when the opportunity to enjoy them is absent. For example, my husband and I were away last fall going to school in St. Louis, and student life kept me very tied to the books. In order to keep up with the reading, tests, and papers, I had to squelch most of my caregiving ideas. When we came home for a long break at Christmas, a day came for helping my son and daughter-in-law with some practicalities. They were both sick and needed some food and housecleaning help. I made a big pot of soup, delivered some to my neighbor who's a widower, and took the rest to Sam and Meg. As I was cooking the soup and preparing to go, I burst into tears of gratitude to God. Those months away from home had frustrated something deep inside me, and now I was able to act instead of suppressing my inner urgings. I could be most fully who I am and feel the satisfaction of it.

We are most content when what we do matches who we are. My friend Judi, an English teacher and drama instructor, knows she's been created to teach and feels satisfied to the bone when she's in front of a class. Another friend, Michelle, is a gifted Bible teacher. She brightens up a room with her passion as she opens the Word for others. The world wouldn't be the same if these two didn't give with the gifts and talents God gave them to use in his service. The same is true for me.

This doesn't mean that our calling will always be easy. We're responsible to care for the people in our families and extended families whether or not we feel inspired to do so. What that care looks like will be different in each case, but we don't have the option of writing each other off no matter how much we'd like to. In my own life, I have one relationship that has been extremely difficult and hurtful. Some days I hit a wall and want to give up. I've had to decide that it's okay at these times to take a vacation from the person, to lick my wounds, pray, and wait on God. What I'm not free to do is wipe that person out of my life forever. I'm called to hang in for the long term, even if it's from a distance—watching, waiting, praying for change in my own heart, doing the deep soul work that's necessary, and hoping for God's good work in both of us. The fact that living out my call can sometimes be hard doesn't mean I can say no to the calling as a whole. It means that I am more reliant than ever on God to do in me what I can't do myself: to extend grace to another human being. And when I entrust my calling to God alone, I know a joy that is even deeper than the delight of results I can see.

As we exercise dominion in God's world, our work will consist of a multitude of callings to serve God in every sphere and stratum of life. The diversity of vocation is enormous, each one necessary for serving the complexity of human need. Our experience of God's lavish love and grace calls us to give away what's been given so freely to us. Through our sacrifice of time, gifts of beauty, and creativity in caring, we are responding to our first call to follow Christ through loving others.

THREE

AGAINST THE FLOW

The Inefficiency of Care

Are we living lives that are good, in some large sense? Lives that contribute to the well being of other people, close at hand and far away, and to our own well being? Lives that are attuned to the good of creation and to the active presence of God?

—DOROTHY C. BASS, *Receiving the Day*

In the summer of 1997 I visited England with my husband and son. At one point on our trip, a friend drove us from London to Bath, and while we were driving through the English countryside, he told us stories of his childhood in Scotland. He said something very simple, yet it stuck with me because it pointed out a universal longing of the human heart. He told us that his years in Scotland were the best years of his life because "people had time for you then."

If there's one thing that characterizes our modern world, it's that people *don't* have time for each other. We rush from one activity to the next; we're overcommitted, overscheduled, frenzied, and worn out.

Many of our time pressures come from outside sources and are not within our control. The long hours required of corporate workers, the travel and the deadlines that factor into certain careers, the hours of home-work loaded onto our children—all of these demands come from systems and decisions made by someone else. But we also normalize frantic life-styles when we don't need to. Whether we take a job that requires a long commute, sign our children up for too many extracurricular activities, or take on more projects and commitments than we can handle, our decisions have long-range consequences that we need to consider. Even when we are the ones who made the series of choices that got us into our schedule crunch, we often feel that our schedule controls us. We yield to the pattern of continual intensity without offering any resistance. We have a grow-ing realization that overcommitment and overwork are destructive, but in general, we don't seem to change.

And as we give in to the standards society sets for us, we gradually internalize what our culture values: efficiency, speed, control, and quantity over quality. In this paradigm, caregiving seems very much out of place. Caring does not "maximize" our time. Its richest rewards are not tangible. Its results are not quantitative. Caregiving needs are unpredictable, and sometimes meeting them is a slow process.

WHAT MATTERS MOST

The busyness syndrome is not new—nor is the way it keeps us from car-ing effectively. Certainly it has been a struggle, in different forms, since the Fall. In recent years, however, the Internet and other technological advances have increased our desire and ability to be very busy all the time.

I first started noting in my journals in the late 1980s how we seemed to be taking more pride in busyness, boasting about our full schedules. We were beginning to believe that activity and having too much on our plates made us valuable. It was happening to everyone, not just people on the fast track in corporate careers. I had school-age children, the responsibilities of family self-employment, and full responsibility for running our home. I felt the constant tug to do more in the schools, in our church, and in the variety of activities my kids were involved in. Those places never had enough help, so I always felt the pull to lend a hand.

I tried to take on the extra tasks carefully, budgeting my time around the rest of my responsibilities. I was still able to tend to relationships with neighbors and friends and care for my family in a thorough way.

Seven years later I wasn't able to make that claim anymore. I didn't know it at the time, but I was on the verge of a lifelong struggle with schedules, balance, boundaries, and commitment. As you'll see, scenes from my own journey reflect the truth that if we are busy beyond the scope of our call—even if we are busy with good things—our caregiving passions and abilities can suffer.

Angles of Life

In 1989 we moved from California to Nashville, where we purchased a home in a friendly suburb. One year later we purchased a then eighty-year-old country church to host a hospitality and teaching ministry called the Art House. The Art House was birthed as a place for people to gather, to develop their minds, and to learn to apply biblical thinking to all of life, with an emphasis on creativity and artistic expression. We also built a recording studio on the church grounds. At first we stayed in our house down the street from the church, but after three years of tending two properties, we moved our family into the church and began the long process of making it our home.

Consolidating all the pieces of our life (home, business, and ministry) onto one property was very helpful. From my office in the house I handled the bookkeeping, tax preparation, and some of the purchasing, correspondence, and administrative work. We operated a little bit like a family farm, with paid work and family work and life coexisting.

Our setup was ideal in many ways. A record producer's life involves long, late hours. Having our studio and home on the same property enabled us to have a closer family life than would otherwise have been possible. We ate dinner together every night and interacted throughout the day. Molly and Sam had easy access to both their parents, and they loved being part of the studio fellowship.

In addition to the ongoing record productions and the Art House work, which included hosting a weekly Bible study for more than a hundred people, in 1995 we started a small record label called re:think. The record label mission was to develop artists of faith who could serve the Church through music *and* compete in the mainstream music world. We had a wonderful staff—five employees and one intern—along with those who volunteered their talents and resources for the Art House. We weren't alone in any of it. Yet managing any one of those areas was a full-time job. Between running a household, responding to the needs of teenagers, and living out our ever-present calling to hospitality of all kinds, we didn't have a moment to spare.

Ideas at their conception are exciting and full of possibility, especially ideas driven by faith and passionate concern, which the Art House and re:think both were. But it takes hours and hours of work to make ideas become realities. We failed to examine our pattern of "heaping on" and acted as if we had no limits. As we kept adding to our already full-to-the-brim lives, we got to the point where we had no enjoyment in our busyness, only weariness and strain.

Family Sacrifices

The consequences of our busyness showed up physically, spiritually, financially, and relationally. Chuck experienced frequent illness. The overwork and stress contributed to an immune deficiency problem that resulted in recurring strains of mononucleosis—a one-time illness for most people.

Pursuing spiritual nourishment as a first priority slipped away from us. This was especially a struggle for Chuck due to the rigors of his work schedule. Nurturing a relationship with Jesus through the careful reading of God's Word and attentive prayer was often lost in the madness of "too much to do and too little time to do it in." And the obedience and joy of gathering with believers in all kinds of fellowship was hit and miss.

Managing the financial load was a tremendous burden. We always had a sense of riding the hamster wheel faster and faster, while never getting anywhere. For example, Chuck would produce several records simultaneously for other record companies in order to finance our own record label! This resulted in an increased work load for all of us, yet it failed to quench the insatiable appetite of our overhead.

At the peak of our overcommitted lifestyle, Molly was away for her first semester of college, while Sam, a sophomore in high school, was home. All too often Chuck and I were in a present-but-absent state of mind. We were nearby but were busy juggling all our responsibilities. Our attention was diffused in many directions, making us less and less aware of our children's needs. As parents we were often coasting. Teenagers face so many hard issues, and our children were no different. We were not always in tune with their struggles, and we sometimes failed to offer strong structure, communication, and protection.

Blending business with home affords many more opportunities for a family to interact and be a part of each other's life in the normal course of a day. But with no official quitting time it also presents the temptation to work continually. Working from home in any capacity requires the discipline and faith to have reasonable starting and stopping times. It requires knowing that God has made us to be more than just human work machines.

Ignoring our internal time clocks and our need for rest and play took away from the fullness of life and made it one-dimensional. We were always tired, always feeling pressure and stress, always wearing frowns and furrowed brows. With the large volume of work to handle in so many areas, I often continued at my desk until nearly bedtime. Chuck always had to return to studio work in the evening hours, and he worked for weeks at a time with no weekends off. Those hours were nothing new, but they were increasingly hard to take with everything else we were doing. Sam was gone more and more, which was natural at his age, but his absence also reflected the deficiency of life in our home. Time for our little family circle was hard to come by.

Our marriage also had periods of crisis. Chuck and I had stopped communicating about much of anything except business. Even though we were working in close proximity to each other, we were preoccupied, each within our own spheres, and were giving each other the leftovers of our energy. This way of operating lasted for an extended period and subtly drove us apart so that the oneness in our marriage suffered. We lost affection and warmth, communication and intimacy. Caring for a marriage relationship requires time—and lots of it. Time to be spontaneous; time to be deliberate; time to be creative in loving each other. We had lost that time, and our relationship was beginning to wither.

Our overload affected other relationships as well. The friendships we had as a couple suffered because we rarely took time to nurture them. Our lives were full with the employees and the artists we worked with. When we had time off, we wanted to hide out like hermits. We had no energy left for more people and no compassion for the interruptions of friends in need.

Gradually it hit me. Our house was lacking a heart. It had become a shell that existed for business and ministry to others, but it didn't offer much to the people who lived in it. We used our home for business functions and hospitality of all kinds. We hosted luncheons for retail and media, national sales representatives, and promotion of current recording projects. Artists often stayed with us. We hosted two Art House events for the community in addition to the weekly Bible study. And our home was part of a Christmas Tour of Historical Homes in our neighborhood. But continually preparing the house for events left us with little energy for welcoming the family or Sam's friends.

Chuck and I both finally unraveled to the point where we had to take action to bring about a change. My own crisis of calling and the problems in our marriage caused by overwork collided. We wound up in a counselor's office seeking help to sort everything out. The consequences of continually striving to go beyond our God-given limitations had resulted in a lifeless home, a time-starved marriage, unhealthy bodies and minds, superficial relationships with friends, and a distracted and shriveled attentiveness to God.

ASKING HARD QUESTIONS

As our eyes were opened to our error, we began to look for ways to correct our course. Our family had to make terribly hard decisions to scale back from the overload. We had to let go of things we deeply cared about. The first thing we did was to move our Bible study to another location. Later, we downscaled what we did with the Art House, eventually stopping it altogether. In 1997 we sold the record label. The scriptural principle from Proverbs 23:4—"Do not wear yourself out to get rich; have the wisdom to show restraint"—was a guiding verse for us. Our problem did not stem from trying to get rich; it came from trying to do too many things that seemed good and right, while giving in to a workaholic lifestyle. In the process of trying to be superhuman and showing no restraint, we had worn ourselves out.

Letting go of the Art House and the record label was very difficult for my husband. These were things that he believed in with every fiber of his being. It took him several years to transition through the consequences of these important but difficult choices. But the realization had sunk in that we could only be truly faithful in a few areas at any given time. We started asking questions then that we still wrestle with today: "What kind of life do we want to have, and what choices can we make to move toward it? Where should we focus our energies, and what should we let go? How can we live out our individual and joint callings more intentionally? Is all the complexity of our days truly necessary, or is there a better way?"

In a sense we were asking, "Has our work, including our caregiving activities, become compulsive? Has our busyness become so intense that we are no longer able to care for people out of love and freedom?" As we considered these questions, several realities of caregiving stood out to us.

Caring Is Spontaneous

As Chuck and I looked at how busy our lives had become, we realized that our busyness had kept us from many natural opportunities to care for others. We recognized that people's needs come at unscheduled moments, and we decided that we wanted room to respond to the unexpected, to build time into our lives for spontaneity. If God brought people across our path who were going through a hard patch, we wanted to be available to listen or pray or ask them in for a meal. A hurting friend can't be hushed up when her tears don't fit the day's perfectly timed schedule. We wanted to be able to act instead of letting the moment pass because our lives were stuffed too full.

Caring Is Deliberate

We also made it a priority to be more deliberate about caring for friends and extended family. We came to understand that our callings included faithfulness to friends, nieces, nephews, parents, sisters, and brothers. As Edith Schaeffer has written, "The frantic use of time to 'do good works,' which then leaves no time to care for the needs of a husband or wife, children or grandparents, sister or brother, aunts or uncles, or the wider family is part of what is responsible for the terrible breakup of families."[1]

I once spent an entire day making homemade cutout cookies for a sick relative who lives a long distance from me. Our relationship is a difficult one, and I wanted to send a gift that spoke a deeper message than something I could have pulled off a store shelf. To make the dough, roll it out, cut the shapes, bake the cookies, and frost them was a gift of time and creativity. I wanted to convey that even though our relationship was hard, it was important and worth a lot of effort.

It can be difficult to care for all the people we're connected to. Caring for our friends and family will happen in many different ways over a lifetime, but it will not happen at all if it's not given priority.

Caring Takes Time

In our time-obsessed society it's difficult to realize the value of quiet acts of caring where one hour bleeds into another with no visible result. Sitting with a lonely man in a nursing home or caring for people through prayer is time consuming. My friend Kathi speaks of caring for people in a hospital room: "Human contact becomes so instrumental in a room full of electronic monitors, IVs, buttons and buzzers for medication, schedules and reports. Listening intently for the subtle requests of patients and just holding their hands, letting them feel the caring touch of a concerned friend or loved one is so important." In all of our rushing and overcommitment, this kind of caring gets lost. Speed and efficiency, which are virtues in our society, rarely apply when caring for human life.

Caring Has Eternal Purposes

Most of the time caring cannot be summarized, quantified, or measured. Not much is ever finished. Or if it is finished, it's finished only for a short time. Families and houseguests get hungry again, clean houses get messed up, babies need to be fed every few hours. The most significant results of caregiving cannot be seen with human eyes.

A young mother once told me that when she weaned her baby, she realized that she had given eight hours a day for an entire year to nursing him, and even more when he was a newborn. Without eyes to see more than finished products, we can miss the significance of this special kind of work. Hour after hour of rocking, holding, and feeding a baby might not look like much to some people, but this mother knew better. She had captured a time that could never be repeated in the life of her child. She had given him the gift of herself and in doing so had to let go of the idea that a productive life is measured by a series of completed, visible projects.

When we live in light of the gospel, we view time and people from the perspective of eternity. Even the small things we do to show people they matter can make a difference. We make our offerings, not knowing if our efforts will even be noticed, but knowing that each person matters supremely to God, and *he* notices. We live by faith, not by sight, entrusting the outcome to God and knowing that we're participating in his work of caring for the people he loves. That knowledge fills all of our caregiving with eternal significance.

If we believe the lie that productivity can only occur in the physical realm, we miss so many ways to contribute to the well-being of others. In reality, the time, energy, and talent we pour into other people's lives may be unseen physically but is vivid and real eternally.

Caring Requires Rhythms of Rest

Having house guests almost continually had exhausted Chuck and me—especially me. I was running on empty much of the time and knew that we needed to change our approach to hospitality. From the beginning of our Christian life we had emphasized the importance of hospitality, but we had not accounted for the cycles of work and rest it should include.

The heart of hospitality is being available to others, and precisely for that reason, it can be draining. So it's essential to schedule periods of rest and solitude. Without those times of pulling back, our inner resources run dry and our giving becomes strained and shallow. "Day after day of welcoming strangers, with no Sabbath rest, drives hospitality and its practitioners to distraction," writes Dorothy Bass. "Their welcome becomes unwelcoming."[2]

A Sabbath rest may seem inefficient, but it is essential to giving real care. For us, pursuing wisdom in this area involved taking stock of our past experience and learning from it. We now know that resting from hospitality is a legitimate and necessary part of our ability to continue offering it. We've taken respite in different ways. We took a prolonged break of several years before doing anything else in our home involving large crowds (apart from holiday celebrations) or weekly commitments. And we're still learning that we need Sabbath-seasons without any guests at all. We need downtime, breaks, and periods of rejuvenation in order to return to our calling with renewed vigor.

Caring Means Setting Limits

Hospitality includes planning menus, going to the market, cooking and serving meals, changing and laundering beds and towels, cleaning up after people, and engaging in conversation at all hours. It is real labor that takes up chunks of a day. When hospitality is a major part of someone's life, it needs to be factored into the big picture.

Chuck and I truly desired to have a welcoming household and to give ourselves wholeheartedly to the people who came through our door. But we could not welcome people fully until we recognized hospitality as part of our work and designed our lives accordingly.

In order to be more faithful to this important aspect of our calling, we've tried to keep our schedule more balanced, keeping in mind that saying yes to hospitality often necessitates saying no to something else. Or a period of time with a full work load and other obligations may mean keeping hospitality to a minimum. We wanted to be fully present to a reasonable amount of people instead of being rushed and distracted with a lot of people. One hard but necessary lesson was becoming comfortable with occasionally saying no to a potential guest. We learned that if our plates were too full already or if we were in need of rest and refreshment, it would be more beneficial for everyone involved if we waited for a better time.

Of course at times people need to come regardless of our other commitments. If we waited for a completely open calendar, we would never open our doors. Hospitality is meant to fit in with the whole of God's callings, and we share the realities of life when we come into the dailiness of one another's existence. The difference for Chuck and me involved setting our minds to be better caregivers—less distracted and more purposeful—by trying not to overextend ourselves if we could avoid it.

Caring Comes out of a Rich Relationship with God

I witnessed a transformation in my husband's habits two summers ago, as he was in the last stages of pulling away from this workaholic lifestyle. He began disappearing at odd hours of the day into different rooms of the house with a Bible and a prayer journal. Daily he filled the journal with names of people and their specific needs. Chuck brought those people and their needs before the Father regularly and made notations when there was a change or an answer. I saw an increased sensitivity develop in him as the noisiness of an overextended life cleared away, making room for him to hear the Holy Spirit's directives. Sometimes he would emerge with a new awareness that someone we knew was needy in some way and that we had the means to help. Most of the time he just recognized the importance of his intercession and faithfully kept the appointment. He began to guard that time, to care for people by sowing in the unseen realm where God gives help in answer to the prayers of his people.

We can never underestimate the significance of time that we spend asking the Father to meet the needs of others. It's an essential aspect of caregiving. God is the only One who is able to meet anyone's need in its entirety, and we are terribly remiss if we leave out prayers of intercession. Praying without ceasing is our privilege and calling in Christ, and we can care for people throughout our days and nights in this way. But we need planning and deliberation in order to come before the throne of grace without other distractions. Devoting ourselves to prayer, being watchful and thankful, presenting our requests to God, are foundational to life in the kingdom. Time for prayer is in constant danger of being squeezed out when our schedules make no room for the "first things" of following Jesus.

BEAUTIFUL INEFFICIENCY

As Chuck and I looked at ways to disentangle and rebuild our lives, one key truth emerged: Caregiving is not efficient. It is impossible to keep caregiving within the strict bounds of a tight schedule. It spills over into the cracks and crevices of time. To give care is to be present for people, to build goodness into the invisible places of the heart, mind, and spirit.

A woman I've known for many years recently died of a terminal disease. When we visited her several years before her death, she expressed the painful frustration of being vulnerable and needy in an overscheduled world. She wanted the people in her family to slow down and pay attention to her. She wanted to be cooked for, listened to, and comforted. She wanted to talk about death and have permission to express her feelings. She needed spiritual help—biblical truth and prayer. More than anything, she wanted and needed time with those who were important to her. Though some of her family members truly ached to be with her and did as much as they could, they were caught in the maze of their schedules.

This woman told me something I've never forgotten: "I'm not afraid to die, but I want someone there holding my hand." This statement cuts to the heart of our human longing for embodied love. Others can't always wait for our schedules to be clear. Their need is immediate and profound.

The challenge to consider how to use the time we're given is always before us. Life presents us with a series of one-time opportunities to show people they matter. If we let an opportunity pass, it's gone forever. It's a difficult and continual battle to resist the frantic spirit of the age, but it's worth the fight. The opportunities to love in the name of Jesus come in the dramatic moments of birth and death, but they are also ever before us in the ordinary, daily hours of life. The sacrifice of our time is a gift that tells someone they're valuable. Do we make time to respond to people in our everyday life, to initiate the invitation, to offer the coffee and conversation, to nurture our marriages, our children, and our friendships?

One day over a cup of tea, my good friend Betty, who's older and much wiser than I am, gave me some insightful thoughts about caring. She told me that when she was younger, she made a calculated decision *not* to be someone who constantly took on more than she could handle. She said that busyness sends out a message to people that you don't have time for them. The state of being frantic, overextended, and distracted drives people away rather than drawing them in and inviting them to the refuge of your company. No one is comfortable coming to someone when they feel like an interruption. This fear of interrupting feeds into the isolating trends of our culture where no one wants to be a bother to anyone else.

In a world that so often values speed, efficiency, and change over continuity and relationship, we are challenged on a daily basis to consider what matters most. God invites us to resist the tangled webs of busyness that imprison us and make it impossible to respond in love to the people around us. If we want our lives to reflect the truth that people matter, we must live intentionally toward that end. If we really believe that people are important and that caring for each other is at the heart of our call to follow Jesus, we must thoughtfully and intentionally offer people something more.

FOUR

✕✕✕✕✕✕✕✕

COMING HOME

The Fruits of Hospitality

It takes great artistry to create a home where people will want
to talk to each other; where they will want to linger over dinner;
where they will want to snuggle up with a quilt and a book on a
rainy day instead of escaping to the shopping mall. It takes skill
and sensitivity to design ways to buoy, comfort, and strengthen
the people we love.

—LINDA BURTON, "The Making of a Home"
in *What's a Smart Woman Like You Doing at Home?*

The home-away-from-home that my grandmother offered my sisters
and me during our childhood left an indelible imprint on my mind
and heart. I spent days at a time with her in the summer, when I was sick,
and at any other time I needed care while my mom was away at work.
The moment I opened the screen door and crossed the threshold into
my grandmother's world, I felt surrounded by caring and comfort. She
created an environment of embodied love. Through her physical, personal
acts of nurture, I experienced the steady provision of an active and stable
home with a wise and loving woman at the helm. I learned from my
grandmother's ways that the anchor of a home is the presence of someone
who cares over the long stretch of time.

THE ANCHOR OF A HOME

In the years since I made regular visits to my grandmother's house, I myself have become a homemaker, a mother, and a caregiver. I have worked in my home and outside my home during different seasons of my life. And though my home and life situations are not identical to my grandmother's, I have become increasingly aware of the value of hospitality—the value of a joyful, caring spirit that offers emotional and physical shelter.

Looking back, I see the evidence of a hospitable life that filled my grandmother's home. Her little house on B Street was the base of operations for service to her husband, children, grandchildren, friends, and community. A seamstress, my grandmother operated her business from home. In addition to sewing for her paying clients, she also used her talents as a way of giving to others. She saved my mother thousands of dollars in clothing expenses by making our yearly wardrobes and clothes for special events. She was a patient teacher who taught my sisters and me to sew as well.

Grandma Martha also welcomed us into the shelter of her life through the meals she prepared for us. With daily provisions of home-cooked food, she showed her love first to my grandfather and then to us. Memories of my grandmother always include the food we made and ate together. When it came time to prepare dinner, we chose one of the many recipes clipped from magazines and newspapers and filed away, and set to work. We cut whole chickens into pieces, peeled potatoes, or prepared cookie dough. We talked while we worked, and that was the best part. We talked about the ordinary events of life. We traded tales of her friends and ours. Grandma was interested in people and held in her memory the precious details of their lives. When I spoke of my own life, she treated me with dignity. She always respected my questions or comments, regardless of my young age. Conversation flowed naturally, and a deep sense of companionship grew.

My grandmother's hospitality spilled out to church and community organizations. She knew all her neighbors by name and called on them regularly, offering gifts from her baking and canning labors. Many of her nights were spent writing letters to friends and family who lived around the country. In all her activities, from keeping the household running smoothly to attending meetings, I was welcome to join her.

These simple, ordinary acts of welcome and inclusion by my grandmother showed me that my life mattered, that I was important and dearly loved. Her home was a bright spot when my own home was often stormy and unpredictable. I doubt that she was aware of the gifts she was imparting—gifts of comfort, security, and the opportunity to observe a woman's life lived creatively and in service to others.

THE BIRTHPLACE OF CARE

My grandmother knew that loving people was a lifework. She also knew that relationships don't happen in a void; they are born in a caring environment.

Creating an environment that feeds our need for order, comfort, and nourishment of the mind, body, and emotions takes work. It must be factored into the whole of our life plan. Whether young or old, single or married, we all need a nurturing shelter and an atmosphere for relationships—a place where we can study and create and welcome others.

We are busy people. The assumption that our homes are private havens in which to retreat from the world has resulted in plenty of closed doors and closed lives. The home *is* a legitimate and necessary place for us to pull back from the public world, to be quiet, and to find rest and renewal in order to have the inner reserves for giving again. But if that's all it ever is, we'll miss the rich fullness of the life God intends for us.

For followers of Jesus, hospitality is a lifestyle in which we're called to participate—"a way of life fundamental to Christian identity."[1] As people of faith we have a heritage of hospitality, and it is not an option only for the particularly gifted. Christ has welcomed us into his presence and his kingdom, and we are to imitate him as we welcome others. Many New Testament passages command all believers to practice and pursue hospitality. Romans 12:13, for example, clearly states our responsibility to other believers: "Share with God's people who are in need. Practice hospitality." Hebrews 13:2 widens the scope of our hospitality to include people who aren't well known to us: "Do not neglect to show hospitality to strangers, for by this some have entertained angels without knowing it" (NASB).[2] Although some of us have callings that lead us to practice hospitality more than others, no one is to neglect it.

Chuck and I have found that the art of hospitality is cultivated over a lifetime and refined in small increments. It has become a part of who we are as a family, and I am coming to understand that I will be learning about it for the rest of my life.

A LIFELONG PRACTICE

At the beginning of our Christian life, Chuck, Molly, Sam, and I lived in a small rental house on 57th Street in Sacramento, California. It was a two-bedroom house with green shag carpeting, a tiny kitchen, and walls with improper insulation and a tendency to grow mold. The rooms were furnished with hand-me-downs. Even in its meager state, that little house contained the first truly good memories of our marriage as we began to live for Someone other than ourselves. We found an orphaned cat at the grocery store, brought her home for Molly's birthday, and before long had a batch of kittens. We planted a small vegetable garden in the backyard and flowers in the front. We made friends with our neighbors, ate dinner together around the table, and turned that old house into our first real home. We had a new awareness and gratitude for the gifts in our lives, accompanied by a new desire to attend to those gifts. The love of God that we were experiencing compelled us to share with others.

Our call to hospitality began as we hosted out-of-town musicians who came to rehearse with Chuck. They slept on our couch and awakened in the morning to my little daughter's conversations with her imaginary friends. We'd known some of these men for several years, and they had big questions about the visible change in our lives. We often stayed up until two or three in the morning, night after night, discussing Jesus and the reliability of the Bible and answering their questions to the best of our ability.

With our new involvement in a church, we learned of the need for people to open their living rooms to teachers and students hungry to learn from the Bible. We didn't have much furniture, but we did have plenty of shag carpeting to sit on, so we made it available, and people came.

The next rental house was our first with modern conveniences—a dishwasher, central heat and air, and new wall-to-wall carpet. The house had once been a model home, so every room had a different style of wallpaper. The kitchen had shiny silver elephants, the living room pattern was patchwork quilt, and the master bedroom had metallic gold and silver vertical stripes. It was an aesthetic nightmare, but we were fresh enough from our years of poverty and family breakdown to be mindful of the privilege of living there.

Out of gratitude we shared what we had, shiny silver elephants and all. We had short stints with two people who needed a room and moved in with us temporarily. The musicians kept coming too. They slept in sleeping bags on the floor, on the couch, or on the top bunk in Sam's bedroom. The kids and I got used to stepping over them each morning! In that house I read cookbooks from cover to cover, experimented with menus, and learned how to prepare expandable meals for last-minute dinner guests. Chuck would often call from the studio to see if we had enough food and then bring his coworkers home to join us for a meal. In all these small ways, as natural extensions of our life, our experience with hospitality grew.

Our 1989 move to Nashville signaled an increase in the number of people we hosted. Friends and acquaintances from California, along with our extended family, began to find their way to Nashville on a regular basis. In his musical travels around the United States and Europe, Chuck met people and invited them to our home if and when they ever found themselves in our area. Quite a few people visited us from those invitations, and some became lifelong friends.

Our purchase of the church building and founding of the Art House brought us to a new level of hospitality as we, along with our coworker Nick, learned to manage and serve large crowds of people. We wanted people to gain insight from the teaching there, but we also wanted to create an environment conducive to conversation, the exchange of ideas, and the growth of friendships. We knew that offering refreshments is central to hospitality, so we always provided some sort of food: homemade cookies, hot apple cider in winter and cold lemonade in summer, or sometimes just tea and coffee.

At present, our life of hospitality is in another phase. It's fancier than it used to be. Our home has been renovated; we have an empty nest and plenty of bedrooms. Unless we have an overflow crowd, no one sleeps on the floor anymore. However, had we waited to have a beautiful home and plenty of space, we would have missed out on twenty years of a very interesting life and many, many precious friendships and memories.

Over the years, I've learned that hospitality is both my strength and my weakness. At times I open the door to our home with a large heart, refreshed and ready, with internal reserves for giving. At other times I've offered hospitality kicking and screaming. When I feel pressured and tired from other work, back-to-back company, or tensions in my home, the welcome is not easy to give. I'm sure the verse in 1 Peter 4:9, directing us to offer hospitality without grumbling, is there precisely because close quarters present so many opportunities to grumble! The clash of personal habits, maturity levels, and family backgrounds produces fertile ground for mounting irritations that can become overwhelming. But whether or not I'm feeling personally up to the task, people come, and God's directive to practice hospitality remains.

THE IMPORTANCE OF HOME

When Chuck and I were first married, my thoughts on caregiving were limited to my work as a nurse's aide at Rosehaven Rest Home. The importance of home as a place of caring never entered my mind. It took me years to move past society's assumptions and realize that caregiving begins in the *home*.

In the 1850s, at the height of an ideology that historians refer to as the *cult of domesticity,* it was understood that "history would be affected by the cumulative impact of women creating good homes."[3] Though it's wrong to idealize the home or to see it as the special sphere of women, we cannot overlook its significance for individuals and for society.

Home is not a neutral place. It gives birth to the ideas and attitudes of our culture. In our disconnected and mobile society, practitioners of hospitality offer nourishment to the bodies and souls of their guests. Whether we are single, married, or living in community, hospitality is an important use of our living spaces and our energies. When people spend their days in the cold steel of office buildings or on the run between airplanes and hotels and conference rooms, the personality of a home is healing. It is a warm and welcoming place where weary, lonely, and broken people find solace.

If we view the making of our home as nothing but a list of chores and upkeep, with no larger purpose than providing a roof under which to eat, sleep, and change clothes, we've missed home's deeper meaning. To develop a truer line of thinking, we need to ask, What happens in the context of a home that doesn't happen anywhere else? Where do feelings of security and insecurity come from? Where do we find out if our life has significance and purpose? What stays with us for the rest of our lives, helping to build and shape the people we become? When handled with care, home enables a person or family to move out into the world with deep resources to draw upon: a volume of memories where close relationships were forged through mealtimes, celebrations, special traditions, shared tears and laughter, and the reciprocal experience of caring and being cared for.

For a home to live up to this amazing potential, one person or a team of people must consider the designing, making, and managing of home to be a necessary and legitimate part of their vocation. Good theater does not happen without a director and a set designer, and neither does a vibrant home life. By giving thoughtful attention to the context in which life is lived, we greatly increase the chances that the life stories unfolding in our homes will be good ones. I don't mean that family life will be without sadness or pain, without consequences from sin and rebellion, and without times of questioning and confusion. But I do believe that the resources garnered from a caring home help us weather all that life brings.

Home is an environment where love is experienced in concrete ways, where talent, compassion, and faith are nurtured, where education about a great variety of subjects takes place, where ideas germinate and grow, where interior security is formed, and where character is sculpted. These essential aspects of human life don't just happen. Their cultivation requires the creativity of an artist, the knowledge of a teacher, the organization and management skills of a leader, and the design blueprints of an architect. The making of a home calls for intention, serious thought, and planning.

When the skill, ability, and intelligence needed to create a caring environment are dismissed or underestimated in today's society, we become willing to give up the various pieces that fit together to make a nurturing home. "Domestic outsourcing" runs the gamut from home meal replacements to services that will put together children's birthday parties, send care packages to kids at camp or college, chauffeur children to after-school activities, and provide homework help and comfort over the telephone to latchkey kids. Child-care centers for sick kids are multiplying. Premade, "homey" boxed dinners are perhaps the most popular form of domestic outsourcing. They can be picked up at grocery stores, day care centers, and drive-through restaurants. Or personal chefs will cook in the homes of their clients, providing up to two weeks of meals to be taken from the freezer and heated up in fifteen minutes.

These services all have legitimate uses. As a steady diet, however, and especially when a patchwork of different services is put together, home becomes devoid of any meaning at all, and we, as individuals, families, and societies, suffer great loss.

Things in life that are meaningful take time and effort to produce. But as we continue to adapt our thought processes to and organize our lives around what gives immediate gratification, we become more impatient and unwilling to take the long view of what we're creating. The demanding spirit that wants everything immediately leaves no room for a slow but steady undercurrent that carefully builds good in the human heart and mind.

TRUE HOSPITALITY

The de-skilling of people on the home front and the demeaning of work that is done there has left a hole in our understanding as to why any of it matters. We ought to wonder whether something very significant is lost when outside services are used regularly. Is it more important for these things to be done out of love by someone who cares than by a paid stranger? What do we lose when making a home for the people we love is no longer seen as a great work of design and intent? What's lost when faithfulness in the ordinary, daily needs of life is no longer valued? We lose what is real. And when we completely lose what is real, the reality of home and its meaning vanishes, leaving us with an empty facade, a shell with no substance. True hospitality draws us to embrace truths about what *home* really is.

Home Is a Place to Be Vulnerable

For guest and host alike, home is a place of freedom from performance. Hospitality does not take place in a perfect world. It takes place in the midst of life's realities: the offer of a couch to sleep on when there's no extra bed, scrambled eggs for dinner when the cupboards are bare, and, as my own guests might sometimes attest, the moodiness of a stressed-out hostess who's running on empty and terribly in need of grace.

When hospitality is practiced regularly, romantic notions of entertaining people in a perfect setting disappear. Karen Mains writes, "Entertaining has little to do with real hospitality. Entertaining says, I want to impress you with my beautiful home, my clever decorating, my gourmet cooking. Hospitality, however, seeks to minister."[4]

Mains goes on to say, "The model for entertaining is found in the slick pages of women's magazines with their appealing pictures of foods and rooms. The model for hospitality is found in the Word of God."[5] I love drawing inspiration and practical help from favorite magazines, but the beautiful photographs can be intimidating. They create false impressions of what hospitality should look like. If you have the means, it is indeed a gift to offer people the fruits of your culinary expertise, a beautiful table setting, and a cozy guest room with extra touches that bring refreshment to the recipient. It's *one* way of doing things. But hospitality is missed if we see it only in terms of large houses and full sets of china. You can live in a two-room apartment, a college dorm, or a small house with a mishmash of dishes from a secondhand store, and still offer warmth and availability to others. Hospitality is created with the welcome of open arms and open hearts, not with wealth.

Our willingness to let others see our imperfections and to receive them in theirs opens the way to honest exchange. It's risky. Facades crumble, and we are exposed as the vulnerable, still-on-the-journey-but-haven't-arrived-yet people that we are. But we also are able to offer the grace of a true home.

Home Is a Place to Be Fed

One of the vital functions of a home is to nourish, both physically and emotionally, the people who dwell there. When the art of cooking is not practiced, more is lost than good food. We've been created with taste buds, a sense of smell, and a wonderful capacity for enjoying the wide variety of food God has given us. A meal can be an amazing work of art, savored for its flavor, aroma, and colorful presentation. Or it can be a simple offering that calms the hunger pangs and meets our body's need for nutrients.

In its essence, a meal is a creative act that has its genesis in the mind of someone who cares enough to plan it, gather the ingredients, and labor over its creation. A tangible sense of well-being comes to rest on a home where someone is bustling about the kitchen preparing food that will nourish the body *and* act as the catalyst for conversation.

Shared meals around a common table have many wonderful outcomes beyond simply nourishing the body. They create time for relational bonding through conversation, laughter, and listening to each other's stories. They provide a setting where the deeper needs of our souls—aesthetic enjoyment, comfort, a feeling of belonging, and a sense of security that comes from being cared for—are tended to. For the one (or the many) who designed the menu, went to market, cooked, and served the meal, it is a time of giving, knowing that the giving is not an empty endeavor.

I can't imagine where our own family would be without the shared dinnertimes that were such a daily part of our lives when our kids were growing up. And our refrigerator door would be much less interesting without all the photographs that capture the meal tables of our current lives—meals with our grown kids and new kids by marriage, with our friends, and with extended family.

If our eating experience consists only of fast-food lunches eaten on the run, microwave dinners in front of the television, or home meal replacements gobbled down after a stressful day, we miss out on a great deal of what it means to be human. Wendell Berry hit the mark with his observation, "Our kitchens and other eating places are more and more resembling filling stations, as our homes more and more resemble motels. 'Life is not very interesting,' we seem to have decided. 'Let its satisfactions be minimal, perfunctory, and fast.'"[6]

The continuity of shared meals is a golden thread for nurturing a family as well as an opportunity for the birth of community as we linger over the table with friends, extended family, and strangers who become our friends when we welcome them into our circles.

Home Is a Place of Spiritual Treasure

Proverbs 24:3-4 says, "By wisdom a house is built, and through understanding it is established; through knowledge its rooms are filled with rare and beautiful treasures." The possibilities for creating rare and beautiful treasures in the minds and hearts of those we care for are infinite. Matthew 6:20 also speaks of treasures: "But store up for yourselves treasures in heaven, where moth and rust do not destroy, and where thieves do not break in and steal." Commenting on this passage Dallas Willard writes,

"Of course this means we will invest in our relationship to Jesus himself, and through him to God. But beyond that, and in close union with it, we will devote ourselves to the good of other people—those around us within the range of our power to affect. These are among God's treasures."[7]

Home, by the nature of its physical layout, draws people within close range of each other. Devoting ourselves to the good of others begins with demonstrating love and service to those nearest us. At home we learn to love with the wisdom, knowledge, and understanding that find their source in God. Within the walls of our home, we can invest in people in ways that make a difference for all eternity. Opportunities to express love are continual: a favorite birthday meal, a bedtime story, cleaning the kitchen for the one who cooked, an afternoon snack to welcome our children home from school. These things matter because people matter. These are the ways we show our love and, in small but significant ways, mirror God's love. So often our acts of love are what help people believe the reality of Jesus' love. We can labor with our heavenly Father, filling the rooms of the lives he puts under our care with rare and beautiful treasure that will never wear out.

Home Is a Place of Creative Expression

The intimate nature of a home creates opportunities for the image of God in us to flourish. When we arrange life around the use of service substitutes, we suppress our God-given urges to love our own in tangible, hands-on ways.

As we grow to treasure what God treasures, home becomes an incubator where we create with him, fanning into flame his image and gifts in the people we love. Creative, thoughtful, and compassionate human beings are brought forth as the caring they receive helps shape them. In our home we can reflect the compassionate, caregiving life of Jesus who healed the sick, gave food to the hungry, welcomed little children, and cared about table fellowship and celebrations. The Holy Spirit's work to teach, counsel, and comfort is also reflected when we ask him to enable us to do the same for others. The image of God as artist and communicator is mirrored when we cultivate imagination, creativity, and communication.

We can all be inspired by the endless flow of creative expression that exists in a home where the art of caring is lived out each day. Home is the place where artistic expression is not just for painters or musicians. It's broad enough to include baking cakes, planting gardens, dancing, writing letters, making gingerbread houses, creating traditions, *and* loving people well.

I'm a gardener, and I till the earth to embellish the environment of our home. I plant mainly ornamental plants and work hard to maintain them throughout the year. To some people this might seem like an impractical waste of time, but I've come to see it as a vital part of our life. When I'm standing at the kitchen sink, I look out onto a scene that's bursting with color, form, and texture. Birds and butterflies visit and find food and add to our enjoyment of the natural world. When I walk down the garden path and spot a new bloom just opening, I worship God and thank him for his attention to detail, for the magnificent array of botanical life. When people come to our home to work in our studio or just to visit, I watch their faces change as they emerge from their cars and are surprised by the gift of beauty—azaleas blooming in the spring or the striking color of oak-leaf hydrangeas in the fall. They begin to slow down, to notice the blooms, the shapes, the color, and the butterflies. They are reminded that goodness still exists in this world.

In a household where creative serving is a way of life, it gets passed on to the next generation. That's why we must begin with our own households to rekindle the art of nurturing, serving, and caring for one another. Only then can we hope to pass on the ability to love others with imagination and compassion. Home is the school where we learn that love shows itself in the details.

GROWING UP AT HOME

Above all, a caring home is essential to the nurture of those we are closest to, especially the generations who come after us. Consider this sobering statement:

> Ironically, it is not just hospitality to the "stranger" that is in peril in our society. We are short not only of tables that welcome strangers but even of tables that welcome friends. In a society that prizes youthfulness, the elderly are often isolated from the affection and care of their own families. In many busy families, children find no after-school welcome home, and spouses find little time to host one another over supper. And when we become estranged—separated by grievances large or small, or simply crowded out of one another's lives—we all too often become "strangers" even to those we once loved. Can we move beyond strangeness and estrangement to learn the skills of welcoming one another and to claim the joy of homecoming?[8]

The most important recipients of our hospitality are our family members. Even now, while Chuck and I are in our empty-nest years, our home must first of all be a place of care and welcome for each other. We need periods of sanctuary and privacy for the continuing development of our relationship. When our marriage is nurtured and healthy, we can give to others out of its fullness.

This new stage of life also brings the desire to make and maintain a family home for our adult children and future grandchildren. Having a familiar place for them to come home to, a sense of roots and connection in an ever-changing world, is important to us. Continuity is such a rare quality in our transitory culture that it helps to have some things in life we can count on to stay the same, to endure over time.

My grandmother's house was a refuge for many reasons, but one of them was the continuity I found there. Everything stayed in place as it always had been. The front screen door always opened and closed with the same sound. I could count on the old green pottery cookie jar to be full and resting on the kitchen counter. The sewing machine stayed on its cabinet by the chenille-covered bed, where I would lie down and talk to Grandma while she sewed. This sameness was a comfort when other places in my young life were full of disruption. I want to give this gift of continuity to our own loved ones. So, for as long as we are able, we will work to keep our home a special place for our family.

It is sad to think of generations of children growing up without the memory of a kitchen that's alive with activity and the pungent aroma of good things cooking—gingerbread, homemade soup, peach crisp, roasted potatoes with garlic. Sadder yet is the thought that some children experience the empty feeling of knowing that their birthday party or care package was put together by faceless strangers rather than someone who knew their preferences and lovingly showed it. And somehow the saddest of all is taking a sick child to a child-care center (especially when it's truly the only option). A sick day should be a time to settle into the care of one who loves you, to become the center of attention, and to receive comfort and help.

My mother died when I was twenty-seven, but in the years before her illness, I went home as often as I could to be cared for by her when I was sick. The memory of Nancy Drew books, icy glasses of 7UP, and cold washcloths on my fevered forehead when I was a kid drew me to her tender care even as an adult.

If children never know this kind of comfort from someone who loves them, how can they give it to anyone else later in life? How do they even know how to value such care? It's possible, as one writer states, to "send a signal to children that any act of kindness can be bought and sold, that there is no such thing as a labor of love."[9]

When we fail to take the time to enjoy creative expression, quiet days at home, and lingering conversations around the table, our children feel it. They absorb our frenzied pace and magnify it in their own lives. A twelve-year-old boy commented in *Time* magazine, "Sometimes I think, like, since I'm a kid, I need to enjoy my life. But I don't have time for that."[10]

Children need to experience firsthand what it means to be fed and nurtured with food that loving hands have made. They need to be offered the raw materials of artistic expression: homemade play dough, reams of blank paper, pens and paints, and craft materials. They need books and music and time to write stories and plays and songs. They need time in the kitchen with their hands in a batch of cookie dough. They need the freedom to ask questions and be taken seriously.

If we value great artists and thinkers, people who are compassionate and caring, we must create environments where children can grow into creative, kind, and thoughtful adults who know what it looks like to put someone else's needs before their own.

Chuck and I certainly didn't provide a perfect home for our children, but we've been delighted to see how the seeds of hospitality we planted when Molly and Sam were young are bearing fruit now. Molly and Mark, and Sam and Meg continue to cultivate hospitality in their own homes. They are welcoming and willing to share what they have, and that is the heart of hospitality—the essence of what we long to pass on to future generations.

READY FOR OPPORTUNITIES

Unique possibilities for hospitality come with each stage of life. Years after my Grandma Martha died, my sister and I found a little guest book among her diaries. It illustrates the value of her hospitality as a single woman. It also speaks to the possibilities that emerge when a community of people work together to welcome a stranger.

My grandmother's church created a ministry to soldiers during World

War II. Those who were stationed at the local army base or traveling through town en route to another destination could find welcome and refuge at Hospitality House. Members of the congregation created a homey atmosphere in a room in the church building. They welcomed the soldiers and their wives or girlfriends. Soldiers and their families had a gathering place in which to make friends over cake and cups of coffee. The congregation opened their homes as well, inviting the soldiers and their loved ones over for Sunday dinners, overnights, and weekends, and sometimes even longer stays.

My grandmother married my grandfather in 1945, several years after his first wife, my mom's mother, died. Prior to her marriage my grandma had been a teacher. She owned a small house and made it available to this ministry. Some of the married couples and the women stayed in her house for weeks at a time. Those who wrote in the guest book expressed their deep gratitude for having a home away from home. They spoke of my grandmother treating them with the kindness and warmth they hungered for as they missed their own loved ones. One man wrote, "We shared our thoughts with you because you listened." Still another guest wrote about how much it meant to have someone listen as he told his hometown stories. One of the women wrote that her homesickness was eased by my grandmother's hospitality. Others expressed their gratitude for the interest she showed in their welfare and happiness.

This little snapshot from my grandmother's life teaches me further lessons about the value and meaning of reaching out to others. Simple acts of hospitality—a friendly welcome, conversation over coffee and cake, a listening ear—go a long way. The costly act of opening our door to others "forces abstract commitments to loving the neighbor, stranger, and enemy into practical and personal expressions of respect and care for actual neighbors, strangers, and enemies.... Claims of loving all humankind, of welcoming 'the other,' have to be accompanied by the hard work of actually welcoming a human being into a real place."[11] Just as God cares for us in very personal ways, so we are to love, not in the abstract, but in real, day-to-day, practical ways whatever situation and season we are in.

When we remember that hospitality comes from an attitude of welcome, we open ourselves to an abundance of creative opportunities for shaping a hospitable life. Hospitality often involves the practical help of food and shelter, but it also includes the provision of relational connection. Hospitality can be as simple as making extra food for dinner and welcoming our children's friends to the table or being the one to initiate conversation with strangers at church, parties, or other social gatherings.

Hospitality can also mean sitting with another person over coffee, showing an interest in who they are. The "ministry of presence," as Christine Pohl calls it, is hard to comprehend in our task-oriented world.[12] Spending time with another person, listening, sharing stories, and bridging the gap of our modern isolation requires an eternal perspective. If we are aware of our call to hospitality, we will be more likely to remember that people are more important than finished tasks.

The desire to have a hospitable spirit changes even the briefest encounter on a street corner. Behind the preoccupied face of a stranger, the eyes that stare straight ahead, and the ears that are hooked up to Walkman headphones, is a person we can acknowledge as a fellow human being with eye contact and a greeting. Living with an eye for hospitable opportunities can keep us from charging through the day with tunnel vision, attuned only to marking off the next item on our to-do list or getting to the next meeting on time.

I recently realized firsthand how important it can be to meet someone who has a hospitable spirit. During the first two months of our brief relocation in St. Louis, I was lonelier than I had been in a long time. We had left an established, rooted existence in Nashville and arrived in St. Louis with some lag time between the end of summer and the start of the fall semester. Until school started there was no easy way to meet people, and my need for relationship made itself very apparent, growing daily with tears at the surface much of the time. At that point we were anticipating a long stay in St. Louis, and the thought of being away so long from all I held dear was truly painful. I loved the concentrated time with my husband, but we both ached for the company of our children and our friends at home. There were days when the loneliness was very acute. As I walked around the neighborhood or washed clothes at the Laundromat, I was constantly on the lookout for a friendly face, someone who would make eye contact and small talk. It was rare when that happened, and I realized then how such a small thing can become so important.

In my normal setting, I'm often guilty of being taken up with my own concerns. Most of us are intent on making it through the fast pace of the day and, in all our rushing around, our friendly demeanor and awareness of others gets lost. But as a new kid in town, I was vulnerable and dependent on the hospitality of strangers. It was a good reminder for me.

The command to love our neighbor is open-ended. God gives us no formulas to follow that will produce the right outcome. Each situation will call for a unique response. But always, at its core, being hospitable is the imaginative work of putting ourselves in another person's shoes. From that vantage point, we can think of how we ourselves would want to be treated and then act upon that knowledge.

SEASONS OF WELCOME

As we recognize the value of creating and cultivating a rich home life, it's important to remember the seasonal aspect of hospitality. We can give in different ways at different times of life, according to our circumstances, the demands of other work, our gifts, and our personalities. A household experiencing sleep deprivation from the arrival of a newborn baby, a household immersed in grief or dealing with illness, or a home full of marital strain and family tension needs to take care of itself first.

When my children were young, there were times I didn't think I could face taking care of one more person because the caregiving was already so constant. People who came to us were needy in one way or another. Those who practice hospitality on a regular basis agree that periods of rest, solitude, and spiritual refreshment are essential in order to avoid emotional and physical burnout. A hospitable life is a demanding one.

This reality leads us to the most important aspect of true hospitality: a trust in God and a reliance on his love for us and others. It is God who provides food, time, and energy. Lately, when I've wondered if I had any more energy to spread around, I've been especially dependent on the strength that only God can give. I've started praying for the ability to welcome my guests as Christ, in the tradition of the Benedictines. Their rule states that "all guests who present themselves are to be welcomed as Christ, for he himself will say: I was a stranger and you welcomed me" (based on Matthew 25:35).

I always have new lessons to learn about hospitality. For example, when I began writing this book in the late spring, I pictured myself working in a semicloistered environment, emerging from my writing room only for nourishment, fellowship, exercise, and rest. But God had other plans.

I had no idea the summer would also include a steady flow of houseguests, with two special events thrown in for good measure. Our guests included a mixture of family, old and dear friends, new friends who needed a place to stay while in Nashville on business, and friends passing through town on their way to another destination. We hosted a wedding rehearsal dinner and, most recently, a David Wilcox house concert for eighty people in our community. Callings coexist and sometimes collide. The calling to share our home did not disappear to make way for my romanticized notion of a writer's life. God was drawing me to a deeper trust in his enabling and in his outcomes for all the avenues of our caring and reminding me to be grateful that people loved us enough to come.

We never know what God may be up to. One of my summer guests and I had been estranged for years, and we had been taking small steps to bridge the gap. His visit to Nashville was a huge move forward in our changing relationship. In my mind the timing was not perfect for a visit of this import. I would have preferred a more open schedule. But, as it turned out, it *was* God's perfect timing as he worked powerfully in the unseen realm of the heart. On the last day of our visit, a conversation at the kitchen table led to words of forgiveness and reconciliation that had been twenty years in the making. The welcome into our home and our life set the stage for God to finish the work he had started years before, when, as a new Christian, I began praying for forgiveness in this relationship to become a reality. Making room for the people God brings into our lives requires faith and trust that he will provide what we need as he leads us.

TIME TO HEAL

In J. R. R. Tolkien's book *The Hobbit*, Bilbo Baggins (the story's hero) is on a long journey through mountains, forests, and dark waters. In their journeying, Bilbo and his traveling companions come to rest at the hospitable house of Elrond.

> [Elrond's house] was perfect, whether you liked food, or sleep, or work, or story-telling, or singing, or just sitting and thinking best, or a pleasant mixture of them all....
>
> All of them, the ponies as well, grew refreshed and strong in a few days there. Their clothes were mended as well as their bruises, their tempers and their hopes.[13]

These lines spark my imagination for what a home can offer its inhabitants as well as its guests. The question is, What do people need, and what can we give? Food, shelter, companionship, comfort, forgiveness, beauty, new ideas, a chance to experience the reality of God's love? The possibilities are as numerous as the opportunities God offers us.

FIVE

CELEBRATING THE STORY

A Return to Ceremony

> As a single year circles around the line that is a life, it brings
> many occasions for reflection, remembrance, and renewal. Each
> community or household can gain strength from offering atten-
> tion to these gifted pieces of time.
>
> —DOROTHY C. BASS, *Receiving the Day*

Our family loves a celebration. We value our festive times so much, in fact, that we installed a permanent disco ball in the sanctuary of our church-home! Because of its size, that particular room has been a gathering place for many groups of people on all kinds of occasions, including multigeneration dance parties. The first summer after we moved into the house, our daughter dreamed up an End of Summer party theme. The kids invited a few of their friends, and we invited some of ours. We made food, decorated with flowers from the garden and candles, set up a little DJ booth, and proceeded to have a great time eating, dancing, laughing, and enjoying one another. Since that first dance years ago, we have had many others: our twentieth wedding anniversary, New Year's Eve parties with grandmas and teens and little kids and middle agers making merry together, and, a year ago last spring, an impromptu dance toward the end of our Easter gathering. With forty assorted relatives and new and old friends, we had already feasted, hunted for eggs, played long games of volleyball, and lingered in conversation—and finally, the mirror ball beckoned!

Celebrations and rituals take many forms. As a family we have learned to be deliberate in marking certain days for refreshment, fellowship, mutual support, and remembrance. Seizing a portion of time and setting it apart for celebration brings fullness and color to what can potentially be the flat routine of life. If we succumb to the drone of today's round-the-clock work schedules, we may find that our days have no distinctive shape at all. However, when we stop other activities in order to turn our attention to each other, ordinary days can become extraordinary. Our efforts to create special occasions show how much our relationships matter. A birthday party, for instance, is a way of saying to another person, "We value you. By coming together in your honor with special food, a birthday cake, candles, and singing, we want to show you how much we care for you." Celebration can be an important sacrifice of love and a significant way of giving care.

GOD'S GIFT OF JOY

In our rushed lives, it's easy to get used to quickness and convenience and to forget to cultivate the art of celebrating. We grab a Styrofoam cup of mediocre coffee from the local minimart or gas station, for example, and over time we lose our memory of the slower ritual of grinding the beans, inhaling the delicious aroma of the coffee as it's brewing, pouring it into a favorite mug, and drinking it in quiet contemplation or in the company of a friend. The movement to make all things convenient and efficient leads to a disregard for the cultivation of ceremony and ritual.

When we celebrate, Dallas Willard writes, "we concentrate on *our* life and world as God's work and as God's gift to us."[1] We honor the goodness of God by stopping to savor what he's given us—relationships, music, food, dance, play, and, most important, the gift of himself.

Celebration, in fact, is a spiritual discipline because it is a means of God's grace to strengthen and transform us. Celebrations, along with the other spiritual disciplines such as prayer, study, solitude, worship, and confession, put us in the path to receive from our Lord. Joy is cultivated as we turn from our daily struggles to remember and appreciate the good things in our life, which come from the hand of God. Willard continues, "It is the act and discipline of faith to seize the season and embrace it for what it is, including the season of enjoyment."[2]

The Bible contains numerous examples of celebrations. In Exodus 15:20, Miriam the prophetess led the Israelite women in a celebration dance. Deuteronomy 16 lists three celebrations for remembering and rejoicing in God's work: the Passover, the Feast of Weeks, and the Feast of Tabernacles. Luke 15:11-32 tells the story of a father holding a feast to celebrate the return of his prodigal son. And in a time yet to come, God's people throughout all of history will rejoice in his presence at the wedding supper of the Lamb (Revelation 19:9). The message is clear: Parties are important in the kingdom!

THE LIFE OF THE PARTY

Celebrations reflect both the art and work of caring. Hours and days of planning, creativity, and labor are poured into the events that form the sum and substance of our celebrating. Designing and working toward these special occasions is time spent contributing to the well-being of others, and it should be included in a comprehensive view of the work of caring for people.

In both my natural family and the family I married into, "the California women" have mixed themselves up into one big beautiful combination of female strength and devotion. They offer a wonderful example of how to blend art and work in celebration. Together they attend the ball games, birthday parties, and special moments of each person in the family. When an event is in the making, they labor together for days, weeks, or months, depending on what's needed, and they create wonderful events out of their love and sweat.

Two years ago my husband's cousin got married. For this special occasion Grandma, the aunts, and the nieces banded together and worked for several months at night and on the weekends. They gathered materials, created decorations for the church, table centerpieces for the reception, and pretty little packets of birdseed to throw at the bride and groom as they left for their honeymoon. They set up the reception hall on the day of the wedding and stayed to clean up after everything was over. Right on the heels of that event, my niece Tessa graduated from high school. Again this group of loving women came together on behalf of my sister's family and cleaned, cooked, decorated, and helped host a wonderful party to celebrate Tessa on her special day. With the help and strong arms of the uncles and nephews who are an important part of these events, these women offered the art of celebration to their family.

When I think about my family over the span of many years, I can see that the regular family gatherings, traditions, and celebrations have helped keep us close. The family ties that grow as a result of our family ceremonies weave a web of love and support around the kids in our clan, some of whom have gone through very tough times in their individual families. Through the hands and hearts of the aunts and uncles and Grandma, the young people have a network of encouragers to strengthen and support them as they grow up.

As I've watched the older men and women pour themselves out year after year to the younger members of our family and have been a recipient of their care, I've learned much about what it means to *be* a family. I've learned that through celebrations and family rituals we can become, in Mary Pipher's words, "the shelter of each other."[3]

THE SHAPE OF CELEBRATION

From observing my own family, growing in my awareness of God's call to care, and receiving wisdom from books such as Edith Schaeffer's *Hidden Art* and *What Is a Family?*[4] I realized early in my Christian life that I could imagine for the good of my family. I could put creative thought and labor into the making of our home and the building of our life together. An important part of this work was to design and plan for the special times, for those events that would begin to fill our memory banks and scrapbooks and photograph albums, telling our unique family story and preserving it for the generations to come.

Like all forms of caregiving, celebrations take different shapes at different points in our lives. When our family of four moved to Nashville in 1989, we left behind the support system and traditions of our California family. New traditions had to be created. For the first five years after our relocation, a slow trickle of close friends from Sacramento made the move to Nashville to find work in the music business. Eventually two of our sisters came as well. As soon as the first group of friends arrived, we began holding our Thanksgiving, Christmas, and Easter celebrations together, including new friends who were without extended family.

After we moved into our church-home, our gatherings rapidly grew in size. With its big, warm kitchen and the sanctuary–turned–living room, the church-home opened it arms wide to welcome people in. Quickly we found more and more reasons to get together, expanding the holidays we observe to include Cinco de Mayo (we have fantastic cooks of Mexican heritage in the bunch!), Memorial Day, the Fourth of July, Labor Day, and New Year's Eve. We always share the cooking, we trade houses, and new people in need of friendship and nurture seem to show up at every gathering. Those of us who've been uprooted from our families and their traditions now have a new thread of continuity and history in our adopted hometown of Nashville.

Shortly after my sister Laurie and Chuck's sister Terri and her family moved to Nashville, we began a new family tradition: the Sunday night dinner. With the expansion of our family in Tennessee, we needed a way to be together regularly, especially since we live in different parts of town and rarely see one another during the week. At that time our children were growing up and moving out of the house, so the dinners also gave us a weekly link to them. The Sunday night dinner became a much-anticipated get-together, a time set aside for strengthening our family ties. It was also a night that often included other people—the kids' roommates and friends or people who we knew would enjoy a family setting. After giving ourselves to the cooking and eating, we sat around the table catching up and telling stories, laughing, and enjoying the ease and comfort of being with loved ones. Later, we often played games or watched a favorite television program until it was time to go our separate ways and prepare for another week.

Other traditions hold significance for our immediate family alone. For example, soon after reading *Hidden Art* for the first time, I had an idea—which I will always know as a divine inspiration!—to make Valentine's Day evening a time to celebrate the love within our little family. I posted an invitation in the kitchen, asking everyone to come to a special dinner wearing their finest attire and bearing a love letter for each member of the family, a letter to be read aloud at the end of the meal. At that time we lived in the house with the horrible silver elephant wallpaper in the kitchen, so I did what I could with the humble means available to set a festive table. I bought a red paper tablecloth from the dime store near our house and set out candles and a bouquet of flowers purchased from the grocery store. Molly and I wore dresses, and the boys wore their best shirts and ties. We sat down to a meal of pasta with prosciutto, sugar snap peas and spinach, fruit salad, crusty French bread, sparkling water in wine glasses for toasting, and cheesecake for dessert. After the meal, we gathered in the living room and read our letters aloud and then we spent the rest of the evening playing together and enjoying one another's company.

For the next ten years we kept this tradition going. Our last family Valentine's Day dinner was held the year that Molly went away to college. We found that, instead of becoming less important as the kids got older, these times became more meaningful. The setting changed as we moved to different houses and even to a different state, but the meaning remained. Sometimes we shared the cooking, twice we ate in restaurants, and once Chuck and Sam created the dinner while Molly and I made dessert and decorated. The year we purchased the church, we read our letters from the loft balcony and danced to the music of Marvin Gaye. We celebrated in a variety of ways, but the letters were always central.

Each year as Valentine's Day approached, moans and groans could be heard in the household. The letters had to be written one more time! But every year I insisted, and the family went along, and each year we ended up in tears as the letters were read. The Valentine letters were a way of setting aside one day a year to lavish written words of love upon each other, to encourage and admire, to make formal apologies, and to say wonderful and heartfelt things that might not otherwise get said. This tradition offered our family a unique opportunity to care for one another that we would not have had without intentional celebration.

MAKING MEMORIES

I keep all the letters from our Valentine's Day ritual tucked away in a scrapbook. Whenever I get them out to revisit the memories, I am moved to tears of thanksgiving. The story that's told in them is affirming and life-giving. They preserve a time in our family that will never come again, a time that passed all too quickly. These treasures, these artifacts of love, remind us of those evenings and point us to the close relationships in the present that our past traditions have helped build.

I've learned that keeping records of our journeys is an important part of our tradition. I keep these letters and other mementos because I am an archivist. Through scrapbooks, journals, videotape, and photographs, I've documented the passage of time and kept a record of the history of our family and others dear to us. In all these ways the journey of our life is chronicled. This is one way I can care for others. When we keep archives, we have the double pleasure of experiencing life the first time around and then again in hindsight, with the perspective of time's passage. Anaïs Nin's words, "We write to taste life twice," also hold true when we think of the enjoyment of poring over old photograph albums and scrapbooks.

Future Generations

Keeping the family history is a tradition of caring that goes beyond the present and has meaning for the future. For example, I write in my journals because I have an inner compulsion as a writer to put down on paper what I think, experience, and observe. These writings are private now, but after I'm gone, I'm confident they'll become a part of the family archives handed down to future generations. My words will help the grandchildren and great-grandchildren who come after me to understand what it was like to be a woman of faith in my generation. They will know where I struggled and where I was most satisfied. They will see the evidence and read the details of God's personal care for me and our family. By recording my story honestly as it unfolds, I can care for those who come after me by giving them insight into the lives of their ancestors, connecting them to our story, and thereby helping them understand their own.

Since the beginning of time, people have always had an urge to record life as it was passing—to draw on cave walls, write letters, make up songs, and tell stories orally and pass them on to younger generations. Since we live within the limits of time, we long for ways to freeze the moments of life and hold on to them, to communicate what we experience and observe.

With the exception of my grandmother's diaries, I have very few artifacts from previous generations. As a result I feel a great loss of connection to those who came before me. Knowledge of these people whose blood runs through my veins has become more important the older I get. I want to know who they were, and I long to know the experiences that shaped them. When there is no one left in the family to ask, the diaries, letters, and photos with names and dates written on the back will be especially meaningful. Family artifacts and written words passed down through generations help us see that our lives are lived in a larger context. We come from somewhere, we're going somewhere, and what happens in between is significant.

Great Is His Faithfulness

The history of God's people throughout all generations consists of choices made in response to him as we relate to one another in families, friendships, daily work, and the festive times of which life is made. Our lives are part of a tapestry that has been in the making long before we were born and will continue after we've gone. God has woven each of us into a place and a role in the history of redemption. The photographs, diaries, and scrapbooks in which we chronicle our lives become avenues for remembering God's faithfulness to us and to his plan.

In some seasons of life, time seems frozen in the shape of adversity. The truth of "God with us" grows murky with our current pain. By looking back over our written narratives and the images we've preserved on film, we gain perspective and are reminded of the ways he has strengthened us and changed our hearts or our circumstances. We can echo the words of the writer of Lamentations: "Yet this I call to mind and therefore

I have hope: Because of the LORD's great love we are not consumed, for his compassions never fail. They are new every morning; great is your faithfulness" (3:21-23).

Documenting our histories gives us reference points for remembering the details of God's sovereign and loving care. Deuteronomy 4:9 tells us, "Only be careful, and watch yourselves closely so that you do not forget the things your eyes have seen or let them slip from your heart as long as you live. Teach them to your children and to their children after them." Recalling the many ways God has comforted us in our troubles—tracing the evidence of his movement in our lives and his answers to our prayers— aids us in giving to others from the comfort and care we ourselves have received from him.

INVISIBLE FOUNDATIONS

One of the saddest things on earth is to hear of someone grieving their life choices, having spent the short time they had on things of very little value, at the expense of relationships with husbands, wives, children, and friends. Unfortunately, it often takes a lifetime for people to realize that relationships are extremely precious and must be nurtured in all sorts of ways. We cannot reap what we haven't sown. Where issues of forgiveness and reconciliation have not been dealt with, where gatherings and traditions and celebrations have not been prized, where relationships have not been sought after and treasured, there will be tragic and empty loneliness.

By contrast, intentional gatherings—events and environments we create where relationships can grow—reflect the wisdom of God. Connections we make help push back the isolation, individualism, and privatization so prevalent in our lives today. The continuity of traditions gives us moorings and roots in a society that is increasingly fragmented and fluid, where change keeps coming whether it's needed or not.

When our son graduated from high school, we threw a large party to commemorate the day. I remember getting up very early the morning after, tired from the weeks of preparation, and reading through all the cards he'd been given. I literally wept with thanksgiving over all the connection and support he had, much of it from longtime family friends who expressed that they would be there for Sam in whatever way was needed in the years ahead. These essential connections exist because we've been sharing life with these people for many years. That morning I was reminded afresh how important it is to be intentional about working for relationships, how vital it is to have common memories to share. It was also a good lesson for me of the value of being there for our friend's children and for our nieces and nephews, attending their birthday parties, graduations, school plays, and other important events in their lives.

Rituals and traditions become part of the invisible building blocks that strengthen our families and friendships and leave a heritage for our children and grandchildren. They provide us with a storehouse of memories from which we can draw for years to come. These memories of taste, smell, sight, sound, and touch become our "interior secret, something of time, place, and history. They are patterns of beauty that we can create, and our people will keep them as the place of their heart, the place that they came from."[5]

Favorite recipes, holiday traditions, parties, music, dinners with family and friends—all of these will be reminders to our children and family of having been loved. "We are stockpiling memories for them to use in the years ahead," writes Linda Burton. "We are filling the corners of their minds with sights and sounds and smells that will re-emerge just when they need to remember that somewhere they are loved, whether they falter or flourish."[6]

Our efforts to go the extra mile in working for deep and lasting relationships will bear fruit into the future. We can resist the dehumanizing influences of society by refusing to be one-dimensional, overworked, joy-less people. We can resist the separation of the generations and the rush of life. We can resist leaving little or no space for celebrating, writing letters, or keeping a record of our traditions. And with eternity in view and our feet planted firmly on the soil of God's creation, we can embrace life, its beauty, and the goodness of God. We can love our people with creativity and passion, resting in the confidence that our investment in them and in all of God's creation is work that matters.

※※※※※※※

SIX

THE WORSHIP
OF A LIFETIME

Caring Within (and Beyond) the Church Walls

Worship is a way of living, a way of seeing the world in the light of God.

—ABRAHAM J. HESCHEL, *Man's Quest for God*

As we grow in our understanding of what it means to give care, our understanding of how we *worship* through care will also deepen. My friend Maggie beautifully demonstrates to me the truth of our call to worship God in all of life.

Along with the work of home and family, Maggie works in the field of creative services and interior design. Last spring one of her jobs was to help a client prepare his home for sale. It was a large house and needed new carpeting to improve its salability. In the process of making decisions, Maggie was in and out of the carpet store for several days, working with a salesman she described as a "big man, loud, sarcastic, and intimidating." Through their daily encounters, Maggie found out that his wife was in the last stages of a cancer battle, and he was exhausted. This information helped her understand that he wasn't a scary man after all; rather, he was brokenhearted and filled with sorrow.

On one of her visits to the carpet store, Maggie came with a gift for the man's wife. Maggie's garden was filled with daffodils, so she cut a huge bunch, grabbed an empty bean can and took off the label, decorated it with a paint pen, and wrote on the can "The Flames of Spring." She took the flowers to the store, explaining to the salesman that one of her favorite authors, Christopher DeVink, called daffodils "the flames of spring." She hoped they would make his wife smile. She was slightly nervous about giving the flowers, unsure of how he would react and not wanting him to misread her intentions. Though he didn't know what to do or say at first, eventually he thanked her numerous times for her kindness. He later told her how much the flowers had meant to his wife and that this had inspired him to have fresh flowers for her all the time.

Maggie told me, "I'm so thankful to God for prompting me to be a part of their lives. I don't know anything about them and don't even know his wife's name. But I do know the Lord used that simple can and those amazing flowers to touch their lives in some way."

This act of kindness isn't an isolated incident; it's a way of life for Maggie. Her love of God, love of people, and love of beauty are woven through each day. Maggie leaves a fragrant aroma in her wake as she goes about her daily life, acting on the Spirit's inspiration and imagining for the good of others she encounters.

TRUE WORSHIP

Maggie's story reflects a real understanding of life lived under the gaze of God, where all that we do every day can be true worship. Following God's Spirit will lead us to uncommon ways of bringing blessing to the world.

When we come to faith in Christ and begin to follow him, a new way of living opens up for us, one that is an adventure in loving. Jesus promised that our lives will bear much fruit if we remain in him. The creation of a fruitful life is *his* work in us, born from our living union with him. We are his work of art, and he's prepared good works for each of his children to walk in. The message of the New Testament, repeated again and again, opens a world of possibility: Love one another as I have loved you. Love your neighbor as yourself. Serve one another in love. Bear with one another in love. Be imitators of God, as dearly loved children, and live a life of love. Look not only to your own interests, but also to the interests of others.

Offering our bodies as living sacrifices to God enlarges our view of work and worship. Work, service, and worship blend together, and false categories for keeping each one separate fade away. The whole of life is our canvas for painting the good story of God's love for humanity. In the words of Dallas Willard, we are "God's creative partner in well doing."[1] When the goal is love, almost everything we undertake is filled with meaning.

WORSHIP BEYOND (AND WITHIN) THE CHURCH

So what does living a life of worship mean to the Church? How does true caring happen within the walls of a church building as well as within the body of believers beyond Sunday morning? William Barclay writes, "Real worship is the offering of everyday life to him, not something transacted in a church, but something which sees the whole world as the temple of the living God."[2]

We are called to care for people in the Church and outside of it. We will fail at this calling if we put our caregiving into boxes of any kind. Loving God and loving our neighbor are deeply intertwined and cross all boundary lines of people and place. As Dallas Willard writes,

In God's order nothing can substitute for loving people. And we define who our neighbor is by our love. We make a neighbor of someone by caring for him or her. So we don't define a class of people who will be our neighbors and then select only them as the objects of our love.... Jesus deftly rejects the question "Who is my neighbor?" and substitutes the only question really relevant here: "To whom will I be a neighbor?" And he knows that we can only answer this question case by case as we go through our days.[3]

In the Church, the idea that God is mainly concerned about our religious life feeds our failure to give holistic care. We often speak and live as if our daily life and work (paid or unpaid) don't matter to God, and that only our "spiritual" activities do. With this mind-set, Christians may see the local church body as their only focus of service to God and spend copious amounts of time attending meetings and working in church ministry. But at home, due to a lack of time, people have little or no awareness of the needs of their neighbors or of the members of their own household. Family connections and other relationships are often sacrificed on the altar of "Christian service."

We can be so wrapped up in service to our church or other organized ministries that we miss seeing the privilege and responsibility we have to care over the wide terrain of life. We forget the truth that God reigns everywhere and that we live to him and for him in the whole of our lives. Along with our responsibility to serve God in our local church, we are also called to worship him by caring well for our employees and coworkers, showing kindness and respect to the server who brings us our lunch, and spending time with a grandmother who's in a nursing home.

On the other hand, we can fail to care *in* the Church when we give in to careerism or constant activity that excludes the Church. When we find our identity in a career or in a crammed calendar, we easily succumb to today's 24/7 work patterns, and the time to give care in our local church body will become scarce or nonexistent. As Leland Ryken observes, "The result of the retreat of Christian thinking about work is that attitudes toward work among Christians are not much different from those in society at large. We find the normal quota of workaholics in the pews on Sunday morning."[4] A lopsided busyness in any one area for a prolonged period of time keeps us from loving our neighbor over the whole spectrum of life.

When the dominant views of society or an insufficient understanding of our life under God shapes our ideas about daily life and work, we lose our sense of the importance of care. If the only thing that counts is service in the church or paid work, of what value is the rest of our life? How can those of us who give the majority of our day to caregiving from our homes know that our work matters to God, to his Church, and to society?

Martin Luther wrote, "The entire world is full of service to God, not only the church but also the home, the kitchen, the cellar, the workshop, and the field of townsfolk and farmer."[5] This view of serving topples our neatly defined categories of work as one part of life, service in the church another, and life at home as completely separate from both work and service. The Church is called to recover a biblical, holistic understanding of work, service, and worship.

OUR TRUE IDENTITY

The search for identity and worth, even when it's unconscious, is often what drives us to live the way we do. In our culture we let careers, salaries, and titles define us rather than who we are as redeemed children of God. For the Church to reflect the reality that all of life is worship and that caregiving is an essential part of our lifework, we need to embrace the truth of our identity in Christ.

Many of us have fallen into the trap of believing that money gives work value and busyness gives us worth. A lifestyle of overcommitment and a hunger to find identity through position and financial status have become the devil's tools in keeping us isolated from the kind of community we long for and far away from the grace-filled, strengthening body of believers God intended.

When we allow ourselves to find identity in anything other than Christ, we become inattentive to our Father's quiet voice. We may be acting in the name of Christ—involved in many aspects of church life, helping individuals in the community, committed to professional or lay ministry—but our attention to the King slips away in all our rushing. Time to draw aside to be quiet, to worship God with focus, to ingest the Word of Life regularly, and to care for Christ's people through prayer is lost. Even our desire for such fundamentals in our relationship to God dries up. We end up ignoring our Father or giving him the scraps of our time. We don't seek first his kingdom or hide his Word in our heart, and we don't have time to be transformed by the renewing of our mind. The most important things in life get pushed aside.

The history of the Christian Church is one long story of God's people grasping the meaning of his grace—his unmerited favor—losing it, and then recovering it. We know where our worth comes from, but then we forget it again.

As followers of Jesus we have a bedrock truth for understanding our value. But because we are forgetful people and we hear other messages all around us, we need reminders over and over again until the truth sinks into the core of our being. As Jack Miller said, and my pastors echo, we need to preach the gospel to ourselves daily. We slip so easily from full assurance of our acceptability and worth—knowing that our righteousness has been bought for us by Christ—back to trying to earn a good record on our own. The gospel message cuts to the heart of all our striving.

Our acceptance comes through Christ alone. Trying to earn approval by any other means—our own righteousness, our activity, the recognition of others, job titles, salary, or good works—is a dead-end street. Though we may forget where our acceptance comes from and return time and again to seeking the approval of others, our status before God is firm and unmoving. It's a gift of grace from start to finish. To try and add anything to Christ's work on our behalf is to fall away from grace. Romans 5:1-2 illuminates our new standing: "Therefore, since we have been justified through faith, we have peace with God through our Lord Jesus Christ, through whom we have gained access by faith into this grace in which we now stand."

The Church can invite us to drink deeply of the fact that, once and for all, we are fully approved of in Christ. No amount of activity or striving to be found valuable will add or detract from the value God places on us. We live in *response* to the grace of God, understanding that "the only thing that counts is faith expressing itself through love" (Galatians 5:6). The gospel frees us to a life of worship as we love, not from guilt, but from gratitude. We worship God as we give ourselves away.

OUR TRUE WORK

As the custodian of a *theology of work,* the Church has often missed its opportunity to encourage caregiving as a legitimate vocation, one that has an essential place in God's kingdom. God calls his people to labor in a great variety of settings. A view of work that only values what is paid or visible to the public reflects a small and incomplete understanding of all that God has given us to do. When even the Church fails to make the connection that caring for people takes thought, creativity, time, effort, and hard work, it becomes obvious how much society's ways of thinking have seeped into our own. We are embracing a diminished meaning of work and vocation rather than the biblical meaning God offers us.

We now have the opportunity not only to dignify caregiving by raising it to the level of work but to recognize that it is a work that glorifies God. David Westcott writes,

> Work has an intrinsic value of its own if it's carried out to satisfy a genuine need. Work for the Christian—paid or unpaid—enables us to glorify and worship God, to participate in his work of creation, sustaining and redemption and to use our God-given talents to his service and the service of others.[6]

Such encouragement is a cool glass of water, and caregivers are thirsty for it! We need to know that the work we do, as we love and serve others (often in hidden ways), has great value to God, to the Church, and to the world at large. Each of us has a deep need to know that our lives have meaning and purpose, that what we do with our time matters. As humans made in the image of God, we are designed to work and to find significance in our work. When we fail to recognize or appreciate a type of work simply because it is unpaid, we do one another a great disservice.

The Church can encourage both a caregiving lifestyle *and* specific caregiving vocations by affirming the comprehensive nature of calling: We are called first to Christ and then to secondary callings of work and relationships. God gives different kinds of work to each of us. Service to God includes paid positions, ministry in a local church, and involvement with parachurch organizations, but it doesn't stop there. *We* are the Church—at home, in our neighborhoods, in places of business, everywhere. When we care, we are glorifying God through our work, our effort, our fruit.

God gives us abundant guidance in approaching our work, whether it is paid or unpaid. The Scriptures tell us to work so that we will have something to share with those in need, to be diligent as workers, to use whatever gift we've received to serve others, and to provide for daily necessities. We're to do all our work in six days, keeping a Sabbath day for rest, refreshment, and sacred assembly. For caregivers this is difficult because babies, children, and sick people don't stop needing care on the seventh day. Still, every effort can be made, especially with the help of family or other support people, for rest and refreshment on some level.

What concerns God most about our work are the extremes of idleness and overwork. He strongly warns against idle hands, laziness, unproductive living, anxious striving, and the love of money. In whatever work God calls us to, we are to work with diligence and prayer, with rhythms of rest and of grace for one another.

As Christians we are free from the limitations and stereotypes our culture places on us. We can celebrate and encourage one another in all our gifts without shame or comparison. Moving away from false ideas about work and settling into the truth will help the Church take the lead in returning respect and dignity to caregiving work. It will also keep us away from unnecessary busyness and make us more aware of the simple ways we can embrace a caregiving lifestyle.

CARING FOR THE BODY OF CHRIST

When we affirm the truth that caring is a way of worshiping and glorifying God, our eyes are opened to the needs of our community and our church body. Making room for others is the first step toward alleviating the loneliness that pervades our society, and it begins with our special responsibility to the body of Christ. Galatians 6:10 gives direction to our caregiving, instructing us to do good to everyone we relate to, "especially to those who belong to the family of believers."

Single people, widows, and widowers have told me that Sunday can be the hardest day of the week. While most people go home from church to a family setting, they go home alone. Many have a real desire to be included with married couples, families with children, and groups of friends.

The special needs of older people, in particular, are too often unknown and not addressed. A friend of mine tells me that the older people in her church feel forgotten. They try to make their needs known, but they find it difficult to get someone to listen. They may have been faithful members for years, but when it becomes harder to make it to church on Sunday mornings, few people notice their absence. They need phone calls, visits, prayer. In a word: connection. My friend sums it up: "We just want someone from the church to know we're alive." Several older widows expressed to me their need for conversation and a friendly hug from a man. They tend to spend most of their social time with women and hunger for a friendly male touch and the wide range of conversational topics that come with a gender-mixed setting.

With a little forethought in food planning or even with a spur-of-the-moment lunch of peanut butter sandwiches, you can make a huge difference by bringing people home for a Sunday meal. And including these same people in your regular weekly activities—the children's soccer match or school play, a casual movie night, a new book group—is a way to help relieve their loneliness.

On the other hand, single people can make wonderful contributions to families. Offering free baby-sitting for an evening or creating a special meal for a mother who cooks every night are enormously valuable gifts. Several young single people were close to our family when our children were in their middle years. They gave us respite on a number of occasions by staying with our kids for three or four days while Chuck and I journeyed out of town to nurture our marriage. Those times were important for our relationship and were possible only because our friends made themselves available to us.

Mentoring is also a way of giving care in the church. We often hear of the benefits of mentoring, but those relationships are hard to orchestrate when they don't occur naturally. Church ministry is often specialized and segregated by age: youth, college, young singles, couples, families. We would be able to give and receive care more fully in the church if we kept the various ages more integrated, creating natural opportunities for all ages to mix. Older folks, for example, are an incredible resource to their congregations, but they are often underutilized. People who've walked with Christ for years ooze wisdom from their pores; an ordinary conversation produces nuggets of truth for someone younger to take away. It's important that we let the older people in our congregations know that we value their company, their life experience, and all they have to teach us.

It's also important for the Church to embrace the fact that the art and work of caring is for men as well as women. A friendship between two young men stands out in my mind. At the time, these men were bachelors and volunteers at the Art House. One winter when the flu was making its way around Nashville, one of the men fell ill with a severe case. He had no family in the area to help him, so every evening his friend brought him food, drink, and the comfort of his company. The sick man credited his friend with making all the difference in the world in the loneliness of his prolonged illness. The caregiver in this situation didn't let the fact that he was young and single, or the fact that he was a man, stand in the way of meeting the needs of his friend.

When we recognize the diverse nature of caregiving, the responsibility to give is spread around, and more people are included in the circle of our care. When this happens, we are truly acting as the Church both inside and outside the church walls.

BEING THE CHURCH

My own understanding of a Christian view of caring continues to evolve. Chuck and I have approached our work and our call to care differently through different seasons of life and with gradual steps of growth. Over the years, we've come to understand more deeply and express more fully the truth that we, as children of God, *are* the Church.

At this stage in our marriage, career, and home life, we are often both home during the day if we're not traveling. We usually begin the day in the "sanctuary" part of our home reading the Scriptures and other books related to our writing, seminary studies, or teaching. If you were to peek in our window, you'd see two people seated across from each other, a cup of coffee at each side, and a book or journal on each lap. What looks like lounging to someone else, we know as work. Early on in our Christian life God placed in us a love of reading and learning, and that love has grown to be a part of how we care for others. We love words and want to pursue knowledge in many directions. Accompanying that drive is the awareness that *what we take in* through our studies *will be given away* in everyday conversations and in more formal teaching avenues.

The rest of our days are filled with a variety of activities, each one a piece of the puzzle in our particular set of callings. We spend small and large portions of the day writing. We answer correspondence. We meet with people for various reasons over lunch or dinner or for an afternoon in our living room. During certain months of the year, Chuck works on recording projects in the studio.

Informal mentoring relationships with men and women are an important part of our life. For my husband most of these relationships are with young musicians and artists seeking help and understanding about their vocations or with executive types in his peer group. People willing to share the wisdom of their experience are an asset to the body of Christ and the community at large. Chuck is fully convinced of his responsibility to pass on what he's learned, and he gives hours and hours of time answering questions, troubleshooting, and offering counsel.

Also included in our workweek is the physical labor needed to maintain our home, studio, and property. It's important to be good stewards of what God has given us by cleaning, making purchases for the studio, maintaining the garden, and doing repairs. The creation of a hospitable and artful environment is inspiring to us and serves those who come to our studio and home.

Whenever possible we take turns with the bookkeeping and paperwork related to our self-employment. It's not only practical and necessary to pay debts that are incurred, but we also consider it an act of caring to pay bills on time. We know what it's like to be a musician family waiting for a check to arrive in the mail. Many of the people who provide services for us are self-employed, and our timely payments eliminate unnecessary stress from their lives.

Chuck and I see all the work God has for us under the larger umbrella of calling. So whether we are hosting a group of students in our home, visiting a neighbor, praying, writing songs and books, leading a small group for our church, recording a jazz record in New York, having lunch with someone in need of encouragement, searching for a wedding gift, preparing for a speaking engagement, or cooking Sunday dinner for our family, we're serving, worshiping, and working. Rigid categories of ministry and work fall away. God's love is our motivation. Our life is one of receiving and giving his love in many ways and worshiping God as we offer everything to him.

Our way of being the Church looks the way it does right now because of our season of life and our particular giftings. The words in 1 Peter 4:10 have helped us understand the value of *all* our gifts: "Each one should use whatever gift he has received to serve others, faithfully administering God's grace in its various forms." Everything we have—natural and spiritual gifts as well as material possessions—is important in our service to God. Lee Hardy writes, "The possession of those gifts places an obligation upon us to use them for the building up of the community of faith and human community at large."[7] Both the Church and the world are served to the greatest degree when we exercise the wide variety of our gifts, talents, and abilities.

Every one of us has so much to offer. Chuck and I are well aware that our lives are enriched by the ways others care for us, ways of caring that we could not express as well as they do. As each of us discovers and nurtures our gifts and celebrates the gifts of others in the Church, we see glimpses of what it means to live a life of true worship. Past stereotypes vanish and failures heal, and we move forward in grace to recognize the Voice that calls us to care in the fullness of our identity in Christ.

❈❈❈❈❈❈❈

SEVEN

THE RHYTHM OF OUR DAYS

Creative Caring Through the Seasons of Life

> God dwells in eternity, but time dwells in God. He has already
> lived all our tomorrows as he has lived all our yesterdays.
>
> —A. W. TOZER, *The Knowledge of the Holy*

I write from the perspective of a middle-aged woman who has already experienced many different seasons of caregiving, and I know there are more to come. While the intensive season of my child rearing years is over, I'm now learning to give care as a mother-in-law, a writer, a friend and mentor to younger women, and someday, Lord willing, I will learn the ways of a grandmother.

Caregiving knows no age or physical limits. Even a child gives care as she loves and visits her grandparents and writes letters to her cousin overseas. People who are bedridden from illness may do some of the most significant caring of their lives as they turn from physical activity to the work of intercessory prayer. Ecclesiastes helps me understand the concept of life seasons: "There is a time for everything, and a season for every activity under heaven" (3:1). What I've learned so far is that caregiving responsibilities and opportunities change from year to year. They come as we pass through the painful times of life as well as the joyful times.

As we journey through different seasons of our lives, we become more in tune with our own unique needs as well. We realize that at times we need to receive care ourselves—and that receiving care can be a way of loving as we acknowledge our interdependence on one another.

CREATIVE CAREGIVING

With the always changing seasons of life, we are offered continual opportunities to be prayerful and innovative in our caregiving. Caring for a tiny infant just home from the hospital is drastically different from caring for that same child who's away at college for the first time eighteen years later. You're still trying to uncover the mystery—what will help, what will soothe, what will bring peace to this child—but your methods will be entirely different. Babies' needs are very physical. They need to be held, rocked, fed, cleaned, burped, and sung to. Older children's needs are more mental and emotional: They thought they were ready to go, but now they're not so sure. They're lonely and perhaps confused. They miss home more than they imagined they would and need a little bit of it sent to them. They need your words—in letters, cards, and e-mails. They need the sound of your voice in a phone call. They need care packages filled with homemade cookies and treats, family photos, newspaper clippings from their hometown, or a drawing from their little brother. They need these things often and regularly. The possibilities are endless for helping them over the hurdles. It takes remembering that their need for care hasn't stopped; it has just changed form.

We can never be all things to all people at all times, but we can be intentional about caring for the relationships that surround us in the present. People will come and go from our lives, and our caregiving responsibilities will shift with the years. Our own needs and our ability to meet the needs of others will change, but our ultimate calling to care remains.

Caregiving Later in Life

For people whose lifework is caregiving, later life presents more opportunities for doing what they love. Without the intensity of the ongoing caregiving roles of the past, older caregivers can enjoy more freedom and diversity in their roles.

My mother-in-law, for example, is a widow in her sixties. Her children left the nest long ago, but she still works hard on a daily basis to care for the circle of people who are in her life right now. On countless occasions, she has been the putty filling in the cracks of need for friends and family. She gives practical help to friends and neighbors who are ill or recently widowed. She is there to bring food as well as to share their tears.

On one occasion a newly widowed friend was completely unfamiliar with the workings of the family bookkeeping. Her husband had always taken care of the finances, and she was completely lost. Mom stepped in right after his death and kept the bills paid, coaching her friend until she could handle things herself.

Mom also makes herself available to older relatives who need her help, whether it's a visit, a ride to their doctor's appointment, or assistance with pets and household needs. She helps plan and execute events in her neighborhood of people fifty-five and over. These events bring fun and laughter to the residents and help solidify their community spirit. Mom makes a point of being present at the basketball games, birthday parties, and school events of all the children in the extended family as well. When she comes across someone in need of a mother or grandmother, she opens her arms a little wider and brings them into her embrace.

Mom is very intentional about keeping strong connections with her children and grandchildren who live across the country. Through cards, e-mail, letters, envelopes filled with photos, surprise packages in the mail, phone calls, visits, and gifts that always reflect her knowledge of the individual person, she lets us know that we're the center of her attention even though we're far away. She doesn't let the distance hinder her caregiving, and she finds creative ways to remind us that we are deeply and dearly loved.

Family Caregiving

Recognizing that caregiving comes and goes in seasons has helped our own family be more attuned to the season at hand. During Sam's last two years of high school, we became a homeschooling family. It was a time that called for a particular kind of concentration and availability. I needed a steady amount of energy and discipline to plan and steer his education, but I also needed to be flexible. Other important things were taking place besides homeschooling, and I wanted to remain alert to them. For example, sometimes the great conversations, when Sam opened up and shared what was on his mind, didn't even start until 11:00 P.M.! As a mother whose last child was soon to fly the nest, I cherished those nighttime chats. They gave me the opportunity to see into my son's heart and mind at that stage of his growth, and I didn't want to miss the moment.

Those two years were also a time to embrace our children and their friends with a welcoming home and lots of shared meals. Sam's friends dropped in frequently, and Molly, who was living in her own apartment, brought her friends home for dinner on many occasions. I gave lots of hours each week solely to grocery shopping, food preparation, and cooking. I was able to give myself gladly to the task because my other commitments were at a manageable level. We knew the time with our children at home was slipping away, and capturing what we could was a top priority. Chuck and I hold those times as treasured memories of moments that will never be repeated again in quite the same way.

Sometimes the work of caring for a family requires stripping back to a minimum what you offer to those outside the household. A friend shared that during a season of marital crisis, she focused all her energies on keeping her marriage alive. She took care of her children, but caregiving that went beyond her front door came to a halt. She remembers: "During that time, I sent no baby shower gifts and cooked no meals for people in my church. In fact, my own family ate a lot of pizza. But I did the most important thing I could do for my children. I worked on my marriage, making it possible for them to have a safe place to grow up. I can almost say I rejoice over that time because we are now reaping the fruits of that labor, with plenty to share with others."

A Return to Caregiving

Sometimes we anticipate seasons of caregiving: after our children are born or when we intentionally purchase a home that is suited for long-term hospitality. When those seasons pass, we may assume they are gone for-ever—but life can shift unexpectedly.

Intensive caregiving can reenter our lives just when we thought our lives were beginning to open up in new directions. For many people, the illness of a parent or spouse signifies a return to concentrated caregiving. For others, it's a sudden, unexpected event. A friend talked to me about a situation that completely changed her life.

About a year after taking on an open-ended caretaking role for my chronically [and potentially terminally] ill sister-in-law and her six-year-old son, I realized that I was going through a grieving process. It helped me to recognize that I had experienced a significant loss by entering into this caretaking role. I had lost the future I'd been planning with my husband, and I had lost a large degree of intimacy with him by bringing people into our household. We also lost our "empty nesters" status as we returned to the challenges of raising a youngster. By recognizing my losses and allowing myself to experience the stages of grief, I was ultimately able to arrive at a place of acceptance that considerably altered my attitude toward my role as a caregiver.

The losses that accompany a return to intense caregiving in later life are very real. As my friend pointed out, we must face these losses in order to move toward accepting them. I remember my paternal grandmother dealing with feelings of deep disappointment and grief when my grandfather was diagnosed with Parkinson's disease at age fifty-five. Not only was she faced with the prospect of his suffering, but the rest of her life would be changed as well. The dreams they shared of traveling and enjoying their retirement years would be lost as the disease slowly and progressively turned my grandfather into an invalid who needed full-time care.

Both of my grandparents experienced huge losses over a period of twenty years. My grandmother was used to leaning on my grandfather in many ways. In their family, they shared breadwinning roles, but he was the main caregiver. He was the one who did most of the shopping, cooking, and cleaning. As the illness progressed, Grandma had to take over roles she was unfamiliar with; Grandpa had done so much, and now she had to do everything. Their relationship was turned upside down as their losses accumulated. The side effects of Grandpa's medication and the progression of the disease took away much of his ability to communicate. They lost intimacy. When transporting my grandfather became too difficult for my grandmother, they lost freedom of movement and essentially became prisoners in their own home. They lost privacy when it became necessary to hire outside caregiving help.

I know my grandmother grieved her losses and finally came to accept the unexpected turn their lives had taken. In 1976, when they were both still living, I interviewed her for a college paper and asked her if she had any regrets. She said, "I only regret that your grandpa has to be sick and we're not able to get around and do the things that we want to. But we're not, and I don't think we ever were, led to believe that this life was going to be easy. I guess when you live with a man for forty-eight years, you become one with each other. There isn't much sense in being alive unless you can be together."

My grandparents learned a lesson in caregiving that I only have a taste of at this point in my life: True caring is a choice. True caring sometimes means choosing to be with someone in hardship rather than without them in prosperity. It is loving over the long haul, loving through disappointments, and loving in the midst of losses that may not be redeemed until heaven.

Listening to Our Lives

We all have to listen to what our own lives are telling us. Are you surviving on very little sleep because you're up in the middle of the night with a baby? Are you up late at night, unable to fall asleep until your teenager comes home? Is this a season when the work of hospitality is especially demanding? Are you offering time and energy to a friend who's in the midst of a crisis? If so, be aware of your own reality and pull back from taking on more commitments than you can handle.

Sometimes we reach a season of life when caregiving, combined with other responsibilities, is just overwhelming and that's that. Nothing much can be done about it. When that's the case, we have to dig in, stay steady, and pray for God to give us strength when we feel our weakness so acutely.

A friend who gave care to her elderly relatives, one after another, explained to me the progression of her prayers over a span of time. When more was heaped upon her than she felt she could possibly handle, at first she would run to her bedroom and dissolve in a puddle of tears, thinking no one else cared. Next, she would cry out to God, asking him to change those in her care who were so difficult and full of idiosyncrasies. In her words, she was "whining" to God. Finally, she ended with prayers for help, strength, and blessing, realizing that God would give her added strength as she asked him—and he did.

LEARNING TO RECEIVE

When we are aware of the seasons in our lives, we will also be aware of our own need to *receive* care at times. Many of us, particularly women, struggle with asking for and receiving help. We're used to juggling work loads in multiple areas, and we become very good at it. We're so self-sufficient that the idea of needing others is almost an affront to our abilities!

But isolating oneself in the Christian life is a dangerous thing to do. We're not meant to walk alone. Because we are the body of Christ, with each part needing the others, we create dysfunction when we fear asking for help and settle into the isolating trends of our culture. I have a friend who lives alone and is shy about asking for rides to the airport or for help getting her car to the mechanic. She doesn't realize that her hesitation in calling on her friends for help actually robs us of the joy of serving her and being part of her life. We are created for interdependence in relationships.

John Stott writes, "To love one another as Christ loved us may lead us not to some heroic, spectacular deed of self-sacrifice, but to the much more mundane and unspectacular ministry of burden bearing."[1] Stott goes on to point out that the command to bear one another's burdens assumes that life *will* bring us more than we can handle on our own. We need one another to help carry the weight in times of grief and sorrow, hard passages of marriage, anxieties concerning our children, and confusion over important decisions. We need others to listen, provide careful feedback, and pray when we don't have any words left. We also need help with ordinary things that come up in the flow of everyday life.

Rejoice with Those Who Rejoice

When I read the words in Galatians 6:2 that tell us to "carry each other's burdens," I usually think of coming alongside each other in hard times. But happy occasions can be an equally important time to offer help. This truth came home to me as I experienced the care of my friends in the weeks and days surrounding the weddings of our two children.

Molly and Mark's wedding came just after Christmas almost three years ago. As the time was closing in, our house was nearing the end of a nine-month renovation, Christmas was a few days away, and fifteen of our relatives from California were coming to be with us for the holidays and the wedding. The renovation of our country church had been a labor of love, taking place over many years, and this was the last phase. Four days before Christmas and two days before the relatives arrived, scaffolding was still up, and Mike, our painter, was still busy with the rooms. The wonderfully talented master carpenters who had created so much beauty were working furiously to complete everything on time, but the atmosphere was definitely tense!

My friends Barbara and Diana assessed the need and came to my aid one morning by bringing breakfast and wrapping all my Christmas presents! While I tended to the many details of wedding, home, and hospitality, they sat on the floor of my bedroom and created beautifully wrapped gifts for my family. It was just the kind of help I needed at that moment.

Our lives were even more complex when Sam and Meg got married. Chuck and I were preparing to move to St. Louis in July to be students-in-residence for a semester at Covenant Theological Seminary. In June Sam made the decision to ask Meg to be his life partner. When the kids began planning their wedding, they decided on their family homes as the setting. They wanted a garden wedding at our house and an outdoor reception at John and Ellen's, Meg's parents. They didn't want a long engagement, so they chose a date in October. The only hitch in all of this was that we would be living in St. Louis, and I'm the *gardener!*

My best friend, Maggie, also a gardener, was already planning to care for the yard in my absence, but this new development took the gardening needs to a whole new level! Maggie rose to the challenge and devoted herself to weeding, hauling heavy loads of mulch, and manicuring everything to perfection through the sweltering heat of a Southern summer.

Her service to me didn't stop there. Maggie's caregiving became more elaborate and extensive as she took on the planning and execution of the wedding rehearsal dinner. Meg and Sam requested Mexican food. As we thought and thought about what restaurant to use but were drawing a blank, Maggie offered to give the party herself—a Mexican fiesta. She would have it in her backyard under a party tent; together we would plan the menu and do the cooking, and she would decorate and handle all the legwork. Maggie is an excellent cook (her heritage is Hispanic), she's gifted at creating artful environments and planning large events, and she loves our family very much. It was an offer I couldn't pass up, especially after she convinced me that not only would she be happy to do this for us, but she would *delight* in it. A special evening with wonderful food in a beautiful setting would be an expression of her love for Sam and Meg and the rest of our family.

Full of gratitude, I went back to seminary and left everything in her hands. Other friends helped too. Diana, who was pregnant with her second child, designed and handcrafted the invitations, addressed them, and mailed them. My friend Kathi, a chef who lives in California, helped us plan the menu over the phone, using her expertise to adjust the recipes to serve sixty people.

Maggie checked in with me every step of the way, but she was the one who envisioned the overall design, made lists, researched the best buys on restaurant-sized cookware, and ran all the errands. While she was doing all that, I was free to concentrate on my schoolwork in St. Louis.

Five days before the rehearsal dinner, Chuck and I came home to

Nashville. When I walked into the dining room of Maggie's house and saw all the evidence of her labor to gather and organize everything that was necessary for the party, I wept. The details of her care were everywhere. She enabled me to change from student to mother of the groom without blinking. All I had to do was put on my apron and get ready to cook!

Kathi flew in the next day and rolled up her sleeves for several days of nonstop food preparation. Another friend, Betsy, gave us a whole day of her labor, shredding chicken, chopping onions and cilantro, and washing massive amounts of dishes. After my female relatives from California arrived, they, along with my sister-in-law Terri, entered into the process by baking dozens and dozens of cookies and ironing tablecloths.

The afternoon of the event, while Maggie was busy with table decorations and Kathi was working hard in the kitchen, Diana was helping our cause from the hospital! The baby had come the day before, but still Diana came to our aid. The mariachi band we had hired needed explicit directions to the house. Diana was the only one who could communicate with them in fluent Spanish, which she did from her hospital bed.

On the evening of the rehearsal dinner, all of our senses were engaged as we entered the sights, sounds, tastes, and aromas of Maggie's creation. The old scarecrow from the vegetable garden greeted us at the arbor entrance, dressed in a brightly colored poncho and sombrero. Passing through the arbor, we entered an outdoor garden room, a grassy area surrounded by flower beds, where the mariachi band was playing. From there we walked into the tent, where all the guests were laughing and mingling. The tables were covered with the colorful vintage tablecloths Maggie and I had been collecting for years. They were decorated with large green speckled gourds resembling swans with their long necks bent, red chili peppers, and berry-laden wild honeysuckle cut from the yard. Tortilla chips filled produce baskets lined with purple napkins. The roasted tomato salsa was beautiful in buttery gold, sage green, and cherry red bowls. Candles of all shapes and sizes were everywhere. Molly crafted a menu for each place setting, and we used combinations of our own dishes and silverware. The decorations were inexpensive, festive—not fussy or stiff—and very beautiful and welcoming. Maggie had taken care to put her own stamp on the look of things, while paying close attention to create something reflective of Sam and Meg, who are warm, artistic, and casual people.

The menu was tailor-made and laced with family memories, along with some new recipes that Kathi brought. I'd been serving Pork Stew with Red Chilies and Black Beans to my family for years. (It's flavored with honey, cinnamon, chilies, and cumin, and the recipe comes from Huntley Dent's cookbook *The Feast of Santa Fe*.[2]) We made chicken enchiladas from an old recipe handed down through Maggie's family. Kathi contributed some new ideas. Her fruit salad made from melons, pineapples, jicama, oranges, jalapeños, and thinly sliced red onions—all tossed in lime juice—was surprising and delicious. And her Arroz Verde—rice combined with a blend of romaine lettuce, cilantro, jalapeños, and garlic—provided color and the perfect complementary taste. The menu was completed with homemade chile con queso dip, handmade flour tortillas, and tubs filled with iced Jarritos (Mexican sodas). For dessert we served Mexican hot chocolate and homemade cookies: traditional Mexican wedding cookies, frosted lemon cookies, and chocolate almond cookies.

Maggie, her husband, Dane, and her daughters Megan and Caitlin, along with my sister Laurie, served us dinner. Kathi kept hot food coming from the kitchen. After the meal (which nobody could stop talking about!), the toasts to the bride and groom, and an after-dinner bonfire, the same crew handled the hours of cleanup.

The celebration of our children's impending marriage was beautiful, personal, and festive. The food was amazing. All the details came together to create an evening that will never be forgotten.

That evening the hands and hearts of our friends and family reflected in living color the love of Jesus to us. Many people were involved in the giving, offering their expertise or labor at just the right moment. But most of all I experienced the intimate care of God through the life of my best friend. Parents are used to giving themselves on behalf of their own children—it comes with the territory. But when months of a person's best efforts are given for someone else's child, that's something very special. It's a sacrifice that flows from devotion to Jesus. Maggie's gift was extravagant. She gave months of her time to my concerns with no other motivation than love.

It was extremely humbling for me to receive help from Maggie that just kept coming and coming. At some points I didn't know how I could possibly accept anything else from her hand. But I was reminded over and over that her help was God's gracious provision for a specific time. With a gift of grace, what can you do but humbly receive it and let go of any notions of paying back the giver?

God's Timing

Maggie's extremely generous care for me during my time in St. Louis was born out of the longevity and continuity of eighteen years of friendship. Over the years Maggie and I have helped each other in all sorts of ways. In earlier phases of our relationship, the help given was more ordinary but still necessary—baby-sitting one another's children or watering flowers and feeding the dog when one of us went out of town.

Attuned to the ebb and flow of our caregiving needs, we knew that God's provision of Maggie's gifts during the wedding preparation was unique to that time. Maggie's schedule is different now, and she couldn't handle now what she could then. And I am back at home now, not in need of care in that particular way. But at that time I was open to receiving Maggie's care, and Maggie was sensitive to God prompting her to become an essential part of this important family event.

Sadly, in our busy lives today, we forget what our ancestors took for granted: *We need each other*. We second-guess ourselves before we ask for help or drop in on someone to visit. We wonder, *Will they be too tired? Will my visit be inconvenient?* Many of us have lost even the memory that a visit can communicate love or that being asked to help can be a gift and a joy to the giver, rather than a burden. We assume we are always an imposition. It's good to cultivate sensitivity, and that is certainly necessary for the realities of modern life. But we can carry our hesitations so far that we deprive one another of the joy and privilege of giving and receiving love.

To carry the name "Christian" means that we will grow in the ways of love as God changes us slowly into the image of Jesus. Incrementally, as the seasons of our lives change, we learn to give *and* receive care through the painful times as well as the joyful ones. We find out just how needy we are and how much we have to give others. And we find that there is never a time when we don't need community.

A TIME FOR EVERY SEASON

There truly is a time for everything and a season for every activity under heaven. There is a time when caregiving is for the many and a time when it's for the few. There is a time to care for friends and a time to care for strangers. There is a time to give our children the best childhood we can because it's the only childhood they'll ever know. There is a time to return to our parents the care they gave us. There is a time to give care as a roommate, a sister, a father-in-law, a next-door neighbor, an aunt. There is a time to receive care knowing that we could never pay back the giver. There is a time to give care knowing that our offering will mean personal sacrifice. There is a time to care for one by saying no to many.

Our God, who does not change, offers us many seasons in life. He calls us to be alert to our needs and to the needs of others by first being alert to him. As we respond to his guidance in the rhythm of our days, he will shape our desires and our gifts, and we will delight in the truth that the call to give and receive care fills a lifetime.

✗✗✗✗✗✗✗✗✗

EIGHT

REST FOR THE WEARY

Recognizing God-Given Limits

Come to me, all you who are weary and burdened, and I will
give you rest.

—MATTHEW 11:28

One of the most frustrating aspects of caregiving is our human limitations. Particularly when caregiving is our lifework, we are always
conscious of our inability to respond in the ways we desire and imagine.
Many nights I go to bed with a head full of ideas that have never become
reality: phone calls that weren't made, a card that didn't get sent, specific
help I wanted to give but couldn't. A by-product of writing a book on
caregiving, for example, is that I have to stop so much caregiving, both
inside and outside of my home, in order to do it! As I enter into a new way
to give care—by writing—I have to let go temporarily of other ways I care.
In each season of life I come up against my own finite existence, but somehow I am still surprised by it.

In 1955 Anne Morrow Lindbergh wrote, "The inter-relatedness of
the world links us constantly with more people than our hearts can hold."[1]
We all acquire relationships and acquaintances over time. I have lived in
four cities, traveled cross-country and abroad, and have been linked to

people all over the world through my husband's music career—and my heart is definitely full of more people than it can possibly respond to. In our relationships, we take on the concerns of another person. They make claims on our heart and mind. In varying degrees we become aware of the details of another person's life. With each communication, we learn more about each other. We come to know of birth dates, weddings, illnesses, deaths in the family, and daily struggles. We want to respond when there is need, to mourn and rejoice with others, but the more people we know, the more difficult it becomes just to stay in touch at all. We wonder how we will ever create enough space in our hearts and our days to love as we want to love.

WHY WE ARE TIRED AT THE END OF THE DAY

Since the invention of the electric light bulb, it has become easier and easier to extend the day's work. Our ancestors used sunup and sundown to begin and end their workday, but we don't have to. Now that we have an array of technologies that give us the ability to stay plugged in night and day, we have the illusion of no natural boundaries.

The reality is that our energies are limited to what God has given us. Even though energy levels vary from person to person, everyone needs to rest, play, eat, and sleep. And each person is subject to mental and physical exhaustion when those basic needs are ignored over long periods of time.

Ecclesiastes 3:11 tells us that God has set eternity in our hearts. Perhaps that's why time frustrates us. We're made for eternity, but for the present we live within the limits of space and time. We want to do more than we can, but we live in a universe that runs on a twenty-four-hour cycle, and we have bodies that require sleep. God, in his wisdom and sovereignty, created the world and all those living in it to exist within the boundaries he has set. When we kick against those boundaries, we inherit trouble: illness, lack of joy, neglected and broken relationships.

Caregivers are particularly subject to the dangers of overwork. Because our culture fails to recognize caregiving as legitimate work, there is a cultural expectation that caregivers should take on more and more. Women in particular feel this pressure. My friend Kathi put it this way: "Many women struggle with thoughts of not doing enough when all the while so many people are depending on their gifts of love." Since most of the work of caring happens behind the scenes, in many people's minds it doesn't exist. This lack of awareness results in more requests from more people for more services.

Again and Again

One of the reasons caregiving is tiring is because it is perpetually unfinished work. Much of it is tedious and repetitive. Cleaning toilets, helping a parent to the bathroom throughout the night, washing endless loads of laundry, driving carpools, remembering to give medications, changing dirty diapers, cleaning the floor under a baby's highchair after every meal—all of these tasks must be done over and over again.

When my children were young teenagers, I was so tired of the weekly menu making, grocery shopping, and daily cooking, I could hardly face it. I'd been doing it for many years without a break and was sick of the repetition. Housecleaning was yet another frustration—a continuous effort to maintain order, with most of it coming undone in just two or three days' time.

Caregiving consists of hundreds of details that add up to a big, important picture. But in the repetition and constancy of the daily rounds, it can be difficult to keep in mind the larger story we're creating. Days often run together with very little variety. Karen, a mother of three young children, expressed her feelings: "We know that what we are doing is valuable, but it's so easy to lose sight of the big picture when your days feel lost to dirty diapers, peanut butter sandwiches, and reading *Good Night, Moon* for the hundredth time." It may take years to see the full fruit of our labor, and in some cases we'll never see it in this lifetime. In the meantime, it can be hard to press on and keep on believing that our labor is not in vain.

Always on Call

Weariness for full-time caregivers also comes from always having to be available. If you've ever watched a mother chasing a toddler while others are relaxing at a picnic, you know what I mean. Caregiving, unlike most other vocations, comes without time off or holidays. A few months ago I spent the night in the home of a friend. Her husband is a musician who travels frequently while she stays home with a toddler and a chronically ill baby. Immersion in her world taught me afresh that the joy and creativity of caregiving often compete with loneliness, exhaustion, and discouragement. The tiny amount of time she had to herself after putting the kids to bed was not enough to refresh her before she had to start all over again in the morning attending to their immediate needs. When no one was there to share the load with her, the constant giving was emotionally and physically draining.

Hungry for Affirmation

For caregivers who receive little validation from our culture, it can be particularly difficult when we receive little gratitude from those we care for. One of my journal entries from 1991 bears this out: "With Chuck gone most of the time, Molly often portraying the negativity of a teenager, and Sam right behind her, there's rarely any appreciation sent my way. Without any positive input, everything begins to be rote, and I lose sight of why I'm doing it." Although I do have a grateful family, probably more thankful and more aware of my efforts than most, at times along the way the lack of affirmation from the culture made affirmation at home especially important.

INTENTIONAL REPLENISHING

Any one of these elements of caregiving can lead to burnout. All of them together often make us wonder how we will make it through the day! At times we may feel helpless to make any change in the energy or time we have available, and even though we cannot change the people around us, we *can* do several things to help protect against burnout.

Counting the Cost

As caregivers we need to be aware of the time it takes to be faithful to our caregiving responsibilities. Our society may not recognize how time consuming and valuable caregiving is, so we need to be intentional about recognizing it ourselves.

I've found it a great help to include in my journal the details of my caregiving work. When my children were young I started writing an account of each day. It's a habit I continue. I start with the morning and recapture the whole day, keeping track of the work, the plans, the menus, the people who came through my door—no detail is too small. This helps me keep a perspective as well as budget my time according to what I know about the hours required to care for those entrusted to me. When the work is documented, I'm less likely to succumb to outside voices telling me I should do more. It helps me understand the calling God has given me so that I can be more faithful to it even when others don't understand.

Downtime

Cycles of work and rest don't come naturally in caring work; they have to be built in. Family members can show their sensitivity to a caregiver's need for rest, refreshment, and variety by stepping in and sharing the work whenever possible rather than holding to rigid divisions of labor.

Caregivers long to be recognized for the hours they spend giving care.

If someone you love is a caregiver, don't take that person for granted. Recognize the solid hours of labor that are spent on your behalf. Understand the time spent planning, praying, imagining, creating, and working. Use your imagination to think about what took place in your absence. Show an interest in what your caregiver has been doing and ask about his or her day.

As caregivers, we can be a force to change the way our work is viewed by others. We need to bring dignity to what we do by redefining the words that describe our work so people will know what they mean. Because the work of caring is invisible to so many people, and because caregiving as a vocation has been neglected by our society, we need to bring it out of the shadows and help people understand what we do. When you value what you do and correctly name it as work, respect and appreciation for your efforts will likely spread throughout your family and beyond.

Caregivers can also be more vocal by asking for what we need. Do we need rest? appreciation? help? We can't force any of these things to happen or change the people around us, but we *can* speak the truth in love rather than storing up resentment. And we can be deliberate and creative in taking care of ourselves. We get so used to taking care of everyone else's needs that we forget our own. We need the refreshment of time to ourselves—the fun of going to a movie, taking a walk, having lunch and conversation with a friend, taking a bubble bath, reading a book, or spending time alone with the Scriptures.

An Audience of One

In our line of work, most of us will fall prey at one time or another to the discouragement of thinking that no one cares, no one notices, and no one is grateful—and that nothing we do will ever change that. Feelings of being misunderstood and underappreciated can lurk below the surface much of the time. When we are tired, bitterness and resentment are more likely to take root.

To remain motivated to care, even when our feelings reflect real experience, we need to remember who it is we're truly serving. Colossians 3:23-24 brings the truth back into focus: "Whatever you do, work at it with all your heart, as working for the Lord, not for men.… It is the Lord Christ you are serving." In Os Guinness's words, we "shift our awareness of audiences to the point where only the last and highest—God—counts.… Living before the Audience of One transforms all our endeavors."[2]

HONEST WITH OURSELVES

Perhaps the most important key to avoiding burnout in caregiving is becoming aware of the needless pressures we may be putting on ourselves. We are often guilty of taking on more than God ever requires of us simply because it's the way people all around us are living. We may feel that the more we give care, the more valuable, productive, and helpful we are. We may even think that if we just give a little more, maybe someone will recognize us the way we want to be recognized.

In reality, when we overextend ourselves, we aren't the only ones who suffer. A person who is drained, exhausted, and spiritually empty has nothing left to offer anyone else. Serving others requires a great deal of inner peace that won't be there if we are stretched too thin.

If we push ourselves to give more because we feel guilty when we don't, others will notice. It will be seen in our attitudes, in our weariness, and in the mixed messages we may send about how we want to spend our time. The "poor me" martyr's attitude can creep in without us even realizing it.

When you are a caregiver by nature, it's difficult to hold yourself back from responding to all the needs you become aware of. But we must always consider the finite amount of time and energy we have and what our callings are at any given moment. If your load is full, rest and watch as God calls other people to provide support.

A few years ago, an acquaintance of mine entered a battle with a life-threatening illness. Though we had known each other for years, our paths didn't cross very often. I ran into her one day shortly after she had received the diagnosis. She told me what she was facing and asked me to pray for her. Of course, I was deeply concerned and wondered if there was more I could be doing. But as I heard about her story from others who were more connected to her family, I realized she had a beautiful network of support within her close circle of friends and her church. They were caring for her in creative, practical, and sacrificial ways. At the time, I was carrying a very full load of responsibilities that I knew without a doubt God had called me to. With all that in mind, I took very seriously her request for my prayers. A reminder to pray for her and her family was the first thing that appeared on my computer screen every morning for months.

I considered my intercessory prayer a very important contribution to her support network, and I rested in the confidence that God was surrounding her with others to care for her daily personal needs. Had I been in her inner circle of friends, or if there had been no one else to help, I would have felt a greater responsibility to adjust other obligations so that I could be involved in a more hands-on fashion. I would have known that the extra work was necessary for that season. When it comes to family and close friends, it's usually obvious when we need to drop whatever we can and run to their aid. After all, our primary responsibility is to care for those we're closest to.

Without navigational tools to help us in our caregiving, we are in danger of putting ourselves in the place of God. He is the only One able to care for everyone everywhere at all times. We are in error if we believe that just because there's a need, we're the one to fill it. Sometimes we *are* the one to fill it, and we must pay attention when we know we have what our brother or sister needs (see James 2:15,16). But when modern life confronts us with endless choices of how to give our time, we can too easily split ourselves in too many pieces.

Os Guinness speaks of this fragmentation we feel when the constantly changing menu of options and bids for our time can overwhelm us. He writes that the "character of calling counters the fragmentation and overload at key points and opens up the secret of a focused life in a saturated world."[3] God invites us to understand that he has given us certain things to do, but not all things, and certain people to care for, but not all people.

For years my pastor, Scotty Smith, has been encouraging our congregation to examine whether we're living driven lives rather than called lives. He advises us "to say yes and no in light of our callings." We are all called to give care in some way. But how do we discern what that means for us beyond our primary calling to care for our immediate family? We have to start by assessing our responsibilities and commitments. Is our life full in areas that we know God has already called us to? Can we handle one more involvement and stay true to our current responsibilities? Do we have an opening in our schedule just waiting to be filled? Is the caregiving opportunity an area we're drawn to and gifted for? Are there already people in place to give the care that's needed? Do the primary caregivers need backup people to give them respite? Is there a way we can contribute to a team effort?

People's needs can be overwhelming, but the help offered by family and friends, each one doing their part, lightens the load and builds walls of support. In her book *Traveling Mercies,* Anne Lamott tells the wonderful, true story of a family whose daughter was diagnosed with cystic fibrosis and the friends who circled them with care. Lamott likens the support to an Amish barn raising:

> I saw that the people who loved them could build a marvelous barn
> of sorts around the family.
>
> So we did. We raised a lot of money; catastrophes can be expensive. We showed up. Sometimes we cleaned, we listened, some of
> us took care of the children, we walked their dog, and we cried and

then made them laugh; we gave them a lot of privacy, then we showed up and listened and let them cry and cry, and then took them for hikes. We took Ella and Olivia to the park. We took the mother to the movies. I took Adam, the father, out for dinner one night right after the diagnosis. He was a mess. The first time the waiter came over, he was wracked with sobs, and the second time the waiter came over, he was laughing hysterically. "He's a little erratic, isn't he?" I smiled to the waiter, and he nodded gravely.

We kept on cooking and walking the dog, taking the kids to the park, cleaning the kitchen, and letting Sara and Adam hate what was going on when they needed to. Sometimes we let them resist finding any meaning or solace in anything that had to do with their daughter's diagnosis, and this was one of the hardest things to do—to stop trying to make things come out better than they were. We let them spew when they needed to; we offered the gift of no comfort when there being no comfort was where they had landed. Then we shopped for groceries. One friend gave them weekly massages, everyone gave lots of money. And that is how we built our Amish barn.[4]

This story is a beautiful picture of each individual contributing to the whole according to their gifts and abilities, time, money, and other resources. Everyone gave something, no one did it all, and people in great need were cared for.

TRUTHS TO REFRESH THE SPIRIT

The art and work of caring—whether for the benefit of family, neighborhood, church, or community—includes labor that's often denigrated and referred to as menial. Cooking, cleaning, tending children, or washing the body of a sick and elderly mother-in-law is often considered low, servile labor.

In the midst of repetitive and seemingly mundane tasks, it is encouraging to remember that Christ saw such work as an essential reflection of love. He himself performed what his society called menial work when he washed his disciples' feet—and he told them to do the same for each other. The message to his disciples was always that if you want to be great in the kingdom, learn to be a servant. By Christ's example and his words, we are assured that no act of service is too low or too menial for his followers. In fact, even the smallest act of caring for another human being is an enormous expression of love to God himself.

God has given ample opportunity for each person to serve him in ordinary, daily life. We will miss the significance of this truth if we understand it only in terms of feeding and sheltering the hungry at a downtown mission outreach, as important as that work is. Care for Christ and his people begins at home and moves out from there.

Jesus' words in Matthew 25:34-40 open our eyes to the immediate and eternal value of personal, practical care:

> Then the King will say to those on his right, "Come, you who are blessed by my Father; take your inheritance, the kingdom prepared for you since the creation of the world. For I was hungry and you gave me something to eat, I was thirsty and you gave me something to drink, I was a stranger and you invited me in, I needed clothes and you clothed me, I was sick and you looked after me, I was in prison and you came to visit me."
>
> Then the righteous will answer him, "Lord, when did we see you hungry and feed you, or thirsty and give you something to drink? When did we see you a stranger and invite you in, or needing

clothes and clothe you? When did we see you sick or in prison and go to visit you?"

The King will reply, "I tell you the truth, whatever you did for one of the least of these brothers of mine, you did for me."

God sees our care for those around us. He places a high value on the meals we make for our hungry family, the care we give to our sick relatives and neighbors, the countless drinks of water we serve to our children and grandchildren, and the welcome we offer to people by opening our home. Jesus made it clear that when we provide for others' daily needs, we're giving directly to him. We serve Christ by serving those he loves.

Christ breathes meaning and significance into the whole of our lives, even the tedious, repetitive, difficult places of caring. Referring to this parable, William Barclay says, "The lesson is crystal clear—that God will judge us in accordance with our reaction to human need."[5] Barclay goes on to explain, "Those who helped did not think that they were helping Christ and thus piling up eternal merit... It was the natural, instinctive, quite uncalculating reaction of the loving heart."[6]

I don't think the passage in Matthew is saying that we'll never be aware that God sees our caregiving. Many times it's that very knowledge that keeps us pressing on. Sometimes we are aware of acting out of obedience to Christ, caring out of a loving heart, yet at the same time, being aware that our efforts will someday be rewarded. At other times we are just reacting to a situation, and our only thought is to meet the need at hand. We're going throughout our day giving care as it's needed and not thinking of anything beyond that.

Our motives are always going to be mixed. Longing to be recognized for the hours of labor we spend giving care doesn't mean we are not caring out of love. It is natural to not want to be taken for granted. But when we are, we have the wonderful assurance that our heavenly Father holds our caregiving in the highest regard. Even though we don't receive paychecks or accolades now, there is heavenly treasure to come.

With this in mind, within the limitations of our hours and days we can make significant, eternal contributions by caring for those God loves. We serve in an upside-down kingdom where God is pleased with the small and unseen, with the widow's mite, the mustard seed, and the loaves and fishes. Faithfulness in the little things will make the invisible kingdom bright and visible. It is not for us to strain against the limits and boundaries that God put in place at the creation of the world and called "good." By his power and for his glory, he brings the increase. And because he cares for us, we can cast our anxieties upon him and run to him to find rest for our weary bodies and souls.

NINE

BEYOND BALANCING

Opportunities for Each Generation

There were still children in the world and while there were children, men and women would not abandon the struggle to make
safe homes to put them in, and while they so struggled there was
hope.

—ELIZABETH GOUDGE, *Pilgrim's Inn*

I t would be difficult to discuss caregiving in all its fullness without asking, "How do we balance the need to earn a living with the need to
care for the people we love?" This question touches on so many emotions,
beliefs, and needs that it has become a very sensitive issue. Books, articles,
newspaper columns, and television talk shows are dedicated to the discus-
sion. While it may seem as if this struggle is a new one, in reality it has
always been around. Every generation has faced the challenge of providing food, shelter, and clothing *and* doing the people work—caring for
children, extended family, friends, and neighbors. Though we do face
dilemmas that are particular to our era, timeless truths can free us to enter
our marriage and child-rearing years with God-given creativity and flexibility so that neither sphere is neglected.

DIFFICULT CHOICES

Although there are many possible ways for husbands and wives to divide salaried and caregiving labor, in our family it was necessary for me to be the primary caregiver. My experience as a family caregiver was always changing according to the ages of my kids, the house and city in which we lived, and whether we had guests in our home. The consistent factor, however, was the guarantee of a full day's work.

Since my husband traveled frequently and worked nights, I took care of all the maintenance of our home, yard, and cars. Through the bulk of our child-rearing years, home maintenance included a thorough weekly cleaning, fixing what was broken or scheduling repairs, decorating, painting walls, and making necessary purchases for the household. Keeping order in the yard meant landscaping and creating gardens, mowing, trimming shrubs, and weeding.

I pored over cookbooks, made menus, grocery shopped, and cooked all the meals. I washed the endless piles of laundry, folded the clothes, and put them away. I transported the kids to and from school, baseball practice, play practice, piano and drum lessons, dentist appointments, and friends' homes. I sewed costumes for school plays. I created birthday parties, Christmas dinners, and holiday events for large groups of people. I paid the bills, did the banking, and ran the errands. I did the work of hospitality—changing beds, cooking, and cleaning up. When my children were small, I took care of their physical and emotional needs and guided their days. When they were older, I packed school lunches, made afternoon snacks, took the kids to art galleries and museums, and worked in their schools. In their teenage years and beyond, I worked to make our home and dinner table a welcome place to bring friends. With the addition of self-employment and volunteer work, my life was very full.

Given the time demands of my husband's musical career, we needed my work as a full-time family caregiver, and we also needed my contribution to our business. This was our need when our income was very small, and many years later when it was more comfortable. But it was also what I chose. I *wanted* to give myself to raising our children and making our home and family life. I loved being a mother and homemaker, and I would not have wanted to forfeit those years for anything. There were many other things I could do later in life, but never again could I be with my children while they were growing up.

What I didn't love about those years was that caregiving had to be so one-sided, that I could only rarely share the more tedious, repetitive maintenance work with my husband. The support role weighed heavily on me alone; opportunities to develop other gifts and callings apart from caregiving were hard to come by. Chuck always gave me verbal support, but the practical support necessary to back it up was not there due to his schedule. The possibilities for Chuck and me to serve each other in love in the multiplicity of *both* our roles and callings was squeezed out until recent years.

These are issues we're still sorting through, changing, and growing in. They're complex because they involve personality, family background, biblical knowledge, business structures, and demands specific to different careers. Chuck and I now enjoy a greater balance of support for each other in all of our callings than we ever have before. The tensions we've experienced have driven us to God, and he is faithfully teaching us his truths.

Each family has to work out how to respond to all of their needs in a way that's right for them. Our own experience has made us realize that no matter how different families are, they face the common dilemma of how caregiving and breadwinning can fit together.

COSTLY DIVISIONS

As children, we may have received someone else's care for years but never considered how it all came about. Caregiving can remain a mystery to us until we're faced with the real needs of our own families and have to step up to the plate and get to work. When young couples marry, they give a great deal of thought and planning to their paid careers, but they are often shocked at the intricacies of bringing care and nurture to a home and family. We learn as we go that the creation of a home and the building of a family won't happen magically. It will take our best thought and action.

History shows that every generation has grappled with the demands of breadwinning and caregiving in different ways, but both kinds of labor have always been present and necessary in the blend of human work. As caregiving becomes less validated by society, we and the generations that follow us face even greater barriers to understanding its validity and importance.

In preindustrial societies, breadwinning and caregiving took place together in close proximity. Men and women worked side by side to sustain their households and care for their children and their extended family. Their labor was divided but reciprocal. They were interdependent. Children's labor was also necessary to the household economy. Children working alongside their parents provided a natural setting for religious instruction and the transference of knowledge and skill in agriculture or the family trade as well as caregiving.

As the Industrial Revolution spread into the nineteenth century, a market economy developed and most income-producing work left the home. Separate spheres of responsibility for the sexes emerged. Middle-class homes were emptied of the father's presence, and mothers became the primary caretakers of children.

The split between work at home and in the marketplace has left ensuing generations trying to discover new ways to cope with raising families and earning wages. We're all born into a specific cultural context and have to live, work, and raise families according to the habits and norms of present-day society, while looking to absolute truths and transcendent values that are the same for all time.

Home Alone

I was born in the midfifties, but none of my own upbringing reflected the fifties stereotype of Mom at home and Dad bringing home the bacon. My parents divorced when I was three years old. My mom raised my sister and me by herself until she remarried a few years later and gained another daughter. My mother was employed from the time I was six months old all the way through my childhood. She had a job because of economic need. She worked sacrificially during the day and continued at night when she came home to the "second shift" of housework, dinner preparation, and kids' needs. Thankfully we lived in a small town and my grandmother lived nearby. Grandma took care of my sisters and me quite often on holidays and in the summer when we were younger.

For the most part, however, we were on our own after school. When I was still quite young, I came home and stayed by myself until my older sisters got home. Later when I was older and they had moved out, I stayed by myself after school and most of the time during the summer. My mom tried so hard to keep tabs on us by telephone, but it never worked. With no adult supervision we had ample opportunity to live secretly and destructively. An empty house in the hours after school and during the summer gave us far too much freedom to navigate the waters of the sixties and seventies cultures and the rebellious inclinations of our own hearts. It also left us vulnerable to those who preyed on children who were home alone. I needed protection from situations I was too young to know how to handle. I needed boundaries and household rules to be practically enforced. I needed someone to be more clued in to my school life, to keep track of my progress, and to recognize when I needed help. I needed the shelter of my mother.

My mom, however, was on the leading edge of a huge wave of women who would go through the trauma and struggle of entering the wage-earning work force while simultaneously raising a family. In many ways, the issues she faced were as complex as those women face today. In the beginning and for many years after, her work away from home was literally driven by the need to put food on the table. Later on it would have been possible to live on my stepfather's income, although finances would have been tight in the winter because his work was seasonal. However, by then, my mom had risen through the ranks and was an executive secretary for the president of her company. She enjoyed her job and the people she worked with. She was building a retirement pension and putting away money to put her three girls through college. And I'm guessing that she always had in the back of her mind the memory of the financial pressures that were present in her childhood as well as the economic hardships resulting from her first marriage.

My mom faced real dilemmas. She loved her job and she also loved her children. And although she knew we had troubles, she didn't have access to the mass of research that is now available, which shows that substitute care and self-care for children have not turned out to be neutral choices. They have consequences—for individual children, their parents, and society. As one fifty-five-year-old man, a former latchkey kid, wrote in a letter to the *Wall Street Journal*'s Work and Family column, "I recognize child care is difficult for many families. But asking kids to stay home alone after school is essentially saying, 'Hey, you be your own parent. I have lots of stuff to do.'"[1]

When we neglect our caregiving roles, we experience the sad results. In fact, the hours between 2 P.M. and 8 P.M., when parents are away at work and kids are home from school, are now being called "crime time," the time when half of all juvenile offenses are committed. An unsupervised, empty house also invites first-time sexual encounters and drug and alcohol use.[2] An estimated five to seven million kids are left to fend for themselves while their parents are away. And it begins early in life. One-third of all twelve-year-olds are latchkey kids.[3] Research has linked teen problems ranging from bad grades to depression with the lack of parental attention.

These kids also may be dealing with a lack of attention from parents who stay at home but are not free—financially, emotionally, or mentally—to give their children the care they need. One important reason for this is that some parents don't realize how important care actually is. Our family experienced this firsthand. At times when Molly and Sam were growing up, Chuck and I were both physically present in our home but were not emotionally available.

Even when we face corporate demands, overcommitted schedules, or financial constraints, we are called to find creative ways to care for our families. The well-being of future generations depends on it.

SORTING THROUGH THE POSSIBILITIES

The choices other generations have made for us and the choices we ourselves have made have ushered us into a more intense dilemma of care where cultural, financial, familial, and professional expectations are extremely high and are often contradictory. It can be hard—especially for women—to know how to care best when we have so many options and, at the same time, so many limitations. Ruth Barton writes,

> With increased options comes an increased awareness of the possibility for making mistakes and this awareness can produce real anxiety. On the other hand, more choices also yield increased opportunities for *good* options—options for spending our time, energy, and resources in ways that are lifegiving for us and our world. These new possibilities touch our longing to make a difference and to know that our presence on this planet matters.[4]

Elizabeth Perle McKenna writes of the challenges women face as they try to find their identity in a world where the all-consuming demands of a profession often don't take into account the realities of their lives. These realities include enormous responsibilities to children and family, the desire to nurture friendships and give to the surrounding community, and the need to have a life that doesn't exclude all other interests and facets of being human. Tired of lives devoted exclusively to careers—which are loved but have exacted such a heavy price—women find it extremely difficult to make changes or adjustments. In the process, they lose their sense of identity.

Speaking of her own slow struggle for change, McKenna writes, "Because the value of my life was so deeply tied in to how well I was doing in my career, I couldn't leave it or change it. I was held hostage by success... I depended on something else external—my title, salary, company—to give me the sense of who I was and what I was worth."[5]

McKenna describes a struggle common to both men and women. In our culture, the yardsticks for measuring success are external: money, power, fame, high sales charts, and connections with people or companies that are perceived as important. This is the air we breathe. We need to recognize how temporary such success is and seek to bring a better, finer, lasting truth to our understanding.

FREEDOM TO CARE

The most important thing we can do to make sure that both our financial and caregiving needs are met is to follow biblical guidelines rather than cultural trends or rigid sex roles that don't reflect biblical truth. When we look to Scripture we discover that we have great freedom to carry out our caregiving roles while we provide financially for our families.

The assumption is often made that mothers should do the lion's share of the child rearing, and yet this idea is completely contrary to Scripture. The Bible gives us a clear picture of intimate, long-term care from both parents. The Old Testament is filled with instructions to both parents to teach their children God's Word and God's ways. (Deuteronomy 4:9;

11:19 and Proverbs 1:8; 6:20 offer some examples of this.) Ephesians 6:4 commands fathers to bring up their children "in the training and instruction of the Lord." The verb translated "bring up" has to do first with bodily nourishment and then with education in its entirety.[6]

Not only is the scriptural mandate for both fathers and mothers to teach, train, instruct, and nurture their children, but in a broad overview of Scripture, we find both men and women doing a *mixture* of economic and caring work. The woman in Proverbs 31 is an excellent example of someone doing paid work and caregiving work. Romans 16:23 speaks of the hospitality of Gaius that was enjoyed by Paul and the whole church in Corinth. Both sexes are called to practice hospitality, to care intimately for children, to provide for extended family, and to love and serve the body of Christ as well as the wider world in real, life-supporting ways.

The enormity of the jobs of caring for children and making a living requires divisions of labor, but God has given us flexibility to work things out in different ways in various cultures and eras. No one way is right for all time. "Elaborate rules, roles, and job descriptions for husbands and wives are conspicuously absent from the New Testament," writes Dick Keyes. "The Bible says nothing of who should earn the most money, cook the most meals, balance the checkbook, or change the most diapers. The form that God has given is flexible enough for Christians in many different times and cultures to be imaginative in the way they build their relationships."[7]

Underlying the debate and these dilemmas are the words of Christ to us as his disciples to welcome our child and every child in the name of Jesus. Years and years of teaching, training, nurturing, and embodying the love of Christ cannot be squeezed into cracks of leftover time. With the birth or adoption of a child, parents begin a long-term, time-intensive vocation. Hope for reversing today's destructive trends lies in understanding the supreme importance of the artwork of raising babies to adulthood. It also centers on the joint responsibility of mothers and fathers to raise children and manage their homes. God gives us the freedom to divide labor in families so that the whole gamut of needs is met. What has not been given is the freedom to neglect either area.

NEW TRENDS

Change is in the air for mothers and fathers who are reconsidering how to best serve their families. The Daycare and Latchkey Generations, born after the midseventies, are rethinking whether they want to raise their own children under the same conditions in which they were raised. More fathers are becoming primary caregivers or adapting their schedules to accommodate the income-producing and caregiving responsibilities for both parents. Mothers are expressing a desire to be more home-based than their own mothers were. We are hungry for ways to have financial security and still provide care.

I've had the privilege of looking in the window of several families' stories as they finesse creative solutions for their family life. Our stories are diverse, and no cookie-cutter solution fits every household. Whether we are in a single-parent family, a family that needs both parents working outside of the home, or a family in transition between locations or jobs, we are all called to care for our children in creative ways that reflect our current circumstances, limitations, and freedoms. We need to ask, "How can we, in our family right now, best care for each other given our gifts and circumstances?" In a fallen world where everything from relationships to business systems is marred, this is a difficult road, and we need to be flexible and creative in meeting the financial and emotional needs of those we love.

Double Duty

Some mothers and fathers share both the economic and caregiving labor, each working inside and outside of the home on a part-time basis and adjusting their schedules according to the needs of the family. Although this arrangement is probably the rarest and hardest to come by, it's not impossible, especially when it's planned for early on. I know of one couple, both professional counselors, who work part-time in their practices and also take on large shares of the nurturing work for their children and household. One parent is there when the other is away, and their boys get the hands-on care of both parents on a weekly basis. These people are willing to live with less money for the sake of their joint responsibility to parent their children and the joy of a close-knit family life.

Another couple, friends of ours in the music business, has made some hard choices over the years. They've thoughtfully and prayerfully said no to certain opportunities that might have advanced their careers but would surely have disrupted their family and caused them to miss important events in their children's lives. They're both very involved in raising their children, and they struggle to make choices that won't compromise that priority.

Jody, the father of three-year-old Nathan, works as a freelance graphic designer and photographer while caring for his son at home. Jody says,

> Laura and I adopted our son about two years ago after a nearly three-year adoption process. At the time our son came home, I was the editor of a small monthly newspaper in our town. Because of the flexibility in my schedule, our son came to my office with me. I was able to work from the office in the morning and from home in the afternoon. That lasted about fifteen months. Even though our son was doing all right in that environment, we felt he needed more "home" and "kid" time than "office time."
>
> Last spring we decided that I would leave my full-time position, rejuvenate my freelance projects, and work from home. While it was a difficult decision in some ways, it was financially the most sound. Even now I arrange my schedule according to his. I avoid making

appointments in the afternoons (nap time) and try to find kid-friendly places to meet with my clients. Fortunately my wife has some flexibility in her schedule, so she gets to work from home on occasion as well.

Our son is able to accompany me on many of my client meetings. In fact, his presence is usually a special request by the client. Even today I was picking up materials for a project and the receptionist announced me as "Nathan's dad." Finding the balance between work, home, and son has sometimes been difficult because while I feel a responsibility to my clients, my responsibility is first to our son and his needs. I have found that some days the needs of a three-year-old toddler consume my time, and the projects need to be laid aside. On the other hand, there are days when the independent toddler takes over and he is content to play by himself.

I'm a lousy housekeeper. I'll be the second to admit that. However, I work those responsibilities around our son's schedule and try to accommodate him first. Even though each day is a little different, I try to be flexible to his needs. He's a good little helper when it comes to cleaning up his toys and putting things away at the end of the day. Most of the bigger chores or family projects (such as yard work and garage) are done on the weekends when Laura and I can both watch him.

Creative Finances

For large segments of the population, the best choice—and the only one that works—is for one parent to be the wage earner and the other to be the family caregiver. Most of the time this choice requires sacrifice. It means living on one income in a two-income economy. It means pinching pennies and driving less expensive cars, keeping old furniture for a longer time, and learning to live within tight budgets. It means resisting the consumer mentality of our culture and the constant pressure to want things we don't really need. And it means remembering that even when one parent is the primary caregiver, both parents have caregiving responsibilities that need to be shared.

Having one parent as the family caregiver does not always result in monetary loss, however. Our society expects longer and longer hours from salaried workers in a wide variety of occupations, creating the need for families to hire out even the small stuff that used to be done by family members. We can find ourselves hiring someone to handle the minutiae of our lives: shopping for groceries, picking up prescriptions and dry cleaning, taking the car for maintenance, handling appliance repairs, and purchasing gifts. Depending on the combination of services needed to keep a particular family going, such as a nanny or day-care provider, a housekeeper, home meal replacements or personal chef service, and a gardener, it can be very expensive not to have a family caregiver. A family caregiver can make an enormous financial contribution through his or her daily work and personal expertise. When a family caregiver does for free what would otherwise need to be purchased, a family can save thousands of dollars.

I walk through life with a circle of gifted and creative women who have discovered unique ways to supplement their family finances while still maintaining a strong presence at home. Many of these women have discovered how to keep the fires kindled under their talents, making contributions to the family income while taking care of their families in a very hands-on fashion.

Maggie, for example, is a whiz at living on a tight budget and making it look like a breeze. She goes out of her way to track down the best buys on everything. She finds pieces of old furniture in junk stores and re-covers or paints them to restore them to beauty and usefulness. The skills in design, cooking, and gardening that she's developed over the years bring a dimension of warmth and beauty to her home. She has also found ways to use her gifts and skills in various ways to create extra income for her family. Her creativity in saving money as well as earning it makes her presence and involvement at home possible.

My friend Diana replaced a full-time job working with at-risk children in the school system with a full-time parenting job five years ago. In doing so she never gave up what makes her unique or the many ways she puts her individual stamp on the world. Instead, she reprioritized and made her work as a mother central. As a singer and songwriter, she still plays in public settings, only much less frequently than she used to. She also does vocal work for recording sessions and creates works of art to sell in local venues. Diana tells me,

> The first thing I did was hold a tie to my previous career in prevention (of substance abuse) for kids. I did grantwriting, reporting, and evaluating from home. As our needs changed, I moved to giving voice and guitar lessons at home during nap time.
>
> Later I cotaught Spanish with Jon [my husband] twice a week for an hour and a half. Isadora [our first daughter] came with us. I stopped teaching for two years with the arrival of Carolina [our second daughter]. This summer I taught a summer school Spanish class in my home. Isi sat in on the class, and it was funny to see a seventeen-year-old lean over to get an answer from her! This fall I'll teach a tutorial once a week while Isi is in school and during Lina's nap time. The lesson time is easy; it's the prep that can kill me.

Diana's way of caring most authentically and fully is to fit income-producing activities around the needs of her family, while being very present on the home front.

Michelle is another friend who brought a wealth of talent to her mothering years, contributing financially while caring full time for her family. She's a gifted clothing designer and seamstress who has been clothing her family in artful, original garments for years. She also sews for other people from her home. She supplements the family income by sewing everything from bridal gowns to wardrobes for recording artists to children's clothing, all while working hard to raise three daughters.

Other friends have kept the vocations they had before children came along but have reduced their work hours to a fraction of what they used to be. My friend Barbara is the worship leader at her church. She also arranges and directs the musical productions for Easter and Christmas. She weaves the planning and rehearsals into her week, but she spends the majority of her time caring for her infant son. Another friend, Staci, is a counselor who had a full roster of clients prior to having children. She now sees clients one evening a week after her husband comes home to take over the household. Barbara is also careful to point out that her work for the church is made possible only through the cooperation of her husband, J. C. On weekends and in the evenings, he becomes the primary caregiver.

Two Roles in One

Single parents have the special challenge of covering all the bases without having anyone to share the financial or caregiving load. My sister Laurie is the single mother of a ten-year-old girl, Indira. Along with being a mother, Laurie is working on her doctoral degree, and she earns income through teaching and research work. With such a full load to juggle, Laurie has found that creative solutions to caregiving are a must. She shared with me some of the things that work for her:

I have had to let Indira do a lot of things for herself. I simply cannot do it all, and she has developed great pride in learning to do certain things. It helps me a lot to know that she is responsible for washing her own school clothes and changing her sheets. She also loads and unloads the dishwasher. I cook dinner as often as I can, she sets the table, and we sit down together. She really likes feeling a part of things.

We have a housekeeper now. This past summer I couldn't afford one and spent way too many hours cleaning and being stressed over all the things I had to do. Indira still cleans her room, but everything downstairs gets done for us. That leaves me time to enjoy her and relieves me of stress. I really want her to live in a clean home, with a certain amount of order.

I also try to treat myself in other ways. I get a massage once a month. Every now and then, if I don't have an afternoon class, I go to a movie. Sometimes if I have a free hour or two, I sneak home for a nap, a sandwich, or to watch something worthless on TV. I've realized that taking care of myself is an important part of taking care of Indira.

It can take time to discover the creative solutions we need to best raise our families and perhaps more time to implement them. But God is faithful to our desires as we come to a deeper understanding of what matters most.

Going Beyond Balance

Choosing to care often means choosing to let something else go. As Diana says, "I *am* an example of someone who contributes creatively to the family finances without putting kids in child care. But I am *not* an example of balance. Something always gives. Either the house becomes a mess or I 'phone in' my lesson plans or bills are late. It's worth figuring out, though, because we do need what I contribute. But I am tired."

These last words honestly reflect the physical and emotional cost many people experience as they work out ways to secure a parental presence for their children. Diana's life has been tailored to fit the ongoing needs of the two little girls who've entered her life. I've seen her bristle when someone makes the offhand comment, "It must be so nice to be able to stay at home," as if it were a luxury. She bristles because the loss of a second full-time income has been a real sacrifice, not something that came easily.[8] But Diana and her husband knew the greater sacrifice would have been to forfeit the well-being and security of their little girls by giving them over to the care of someone else. This is how caregiving took form in their lives.

Laurie writes that getting enough sleep is a sacrifice for her as a student and career woman but necessary for her as a mother:

Sleep is the only answer for me in terms of my mental health. I try to always get seven to eight hours of it, even if that means not doing the best on my homework. I've had to let go of my need to be the most prepared student in class. If I don't get sleep, I know I will get sick, and then what good am I?

Sometimes families need to deliberately choose losses for the sake of greater gains in their children's lives. Jody notes,

I can't count the times when at the end of the day I feel that there isn't a single accomplishment that I can point to. Did I finish the dishes? No. Straighten the house? No. Did I finish that client project? No. What did I get done? I read to my son, we ran some errands, and lunch went off without a hitch. Not much to some people, but it has become more and more precious to my wife and me when we can stop and care when our son needs caring.

My wife and I have made the conscious effort to stop what we are doing and spend as much time with our son as possible. Sometimes that means putting off a project until after bedtime or rescheduling a client meeting because he needs to go to the doctor. While these may sound like obvious decisions to some, I believe that the decision to make him first takes some effort. We all want to be "first"; as adults, we have to let go of that and put our children first.

The stories of all these families are examples of the creativity we have in shaping our lives so that our children come first. For many, many families it is truly not an option to have a parent at home during the day. Single parents who are struggling to meet all the breadwinning and caregiving needs and two-income families who need every penny of their earnings need help and compassion from extended family, neighbors, friends, and the Church. This is one of many good reasons for rebuilding networks of unpaid services that friends, relatives, and neighbors can exchange with one another.

For other families the lifestyle that requires both parents to be away from home much of the time is accepted without question. Couples don't give a lot of creative thought to alternate ways of earning income or spending less. In truth, it is well within our realm of power to want less and to resist the notion that we need all that we think we need. We can pray for discernment to learn what drives our spending habits. Is our spending driven most of the time by real necessity or by the consumer mentality of our culture, where shopping and acquiring "stuff" is an accepted pastime?

We are mistaken when we think that kids need an array of electronic gadgets and weekly trips to the mall. One of my sisters just took her daughter on a trip that involved a whirlwind of elaborate entertainment—Disneyland, Disney's California Adventure, and two live theater productions. After all that, the favorite parts of the whole trip for my niece were spending time with her aunts and cousins and swimming. It was a good reminder for my sister and me that what kids love and remember most are the simple things—and the free ones.

WORK-FORCE PRESSURES

The difficulties we currently face in sorting out breadwinning and caregiving dilemmas are exacerbated by the increased hours demanded of people in the paid work force—ranging from factory workers to corporate executives. This was the number one problem in our family and one that we battled, gave in to, and battled again. My husband was a very involved father, but I know he longed for even more time with our kids. We saw firsthand how the long, unrelenting hours of an all-consuming career, if allowed free rein, will eat into the marriage partnership. Difficulties can also arise when one parent is the wage earner and the other is the full-time caregiver. The caregiver rarely gets any relief from the routines and has little or no opportunity to develop his or her gifts and callings apart from caregiving.

After all our struggles, I'm convinced that Christians should be the front-runners in working for reform when the demands of any job or career consistently call for the relinquishing of responsibilities at home. Borrowing from a television interview with Penelope Leach, Mardi Keyes points out that business and industry are dependent on the labor of people who are parents. This fact gives parents far more power to influence the corporate world than they realize. Keyes suggests that parents "can unite and put pressure on companies to institute part time, flexible hours, job share arrangements, day care on-site for part time [employees], and increased maternity and parental leave." In summation, both Keyes and Leach encourage parents to stop allowing industry to play God.[9] When people are asked to serve their careers to such a degree that the other callings of husband, wife, parent, and friend get pressed into a tiny version of what they're meant to be, something is very wrong.

It's an uphill battle to come against an entire system or corporation where long hours, constant travel, and workaholism are expected and accepted. It will take courage and faith, it will mean failure and frustration, and it will require fresh attempts again and again. In many ways, the easiest response is to give in and ride the wave, declaring that nothing can be done. But as in all aspects of life, choices have consequences. It's not uncommon for parents to wake up one day and realize that they've missed most of their kid's childhood and there's no going back.

Os Guinness writes, "Calling introduces into society a different style of operating that directly counters the market mentality. We do what we do in life because we are called to it rather than because we get paid for it."[10] When caregiving is taken seriously as a calling, our minds are open to ways of giving care that may not be obvious at first.

I recently talked with a woman who is convinced that God is calling her to areas of service that are unsalaried. She is particularly drawn to volunteer hospice work. She's married, and her husband's income generates enough money for them to live on. The difficulty is in convincing others of this fact. In order to do the volunteer work, she would need to quit a well-paying job. This is hard for close friends and family to understand.

These are difficult issues to wade through. None of us lives isolated from our culture and its expectations. But God's calling always transcends our temporary social conventions. As we follow him in the unique places he calls us to serve, a world that is falling apart for lack of care will experience significant healing—one person at a time.

<hr>

There are as many creative ways to approach breadwinning and caregiving as there are creative people—and this means all of us, since God has made each of us in his image and given us the capacity to creatively solve problems. Whether we work in the home, outside the home, or both, we have the opportunity to be caregivers because we were created to care.

We answer to a higher authority, One who has made it clear that we are to be about the business of earning our daily bread *and* loving our neighbor, beginning with our immediate and extended family and moving out from there. When breadwinning is allowed to eclipse caregiving and to become the driving force in our lives, the world's system of thinking and doing has won.

We do have hope. Emerging generations can change the drift of society by entering adulthood and marriage with an understanding that both caregiving and breadwinning are part of one larger, holistic work. There are imaginative, creative ways to live so that neither of these areas of responsibility suffers neglect. Developing the art of caring begins with the knowledge that every single person has caregiving privileges and responsibilities: parent to child, child to parent, grandchildren to grandparents, friend to friend, the body of Christ one to another.

People need beauty, continuity, community, inspiration, and real experiences rather than artificial ones. We need to cultivate these in all sorts of ways, to connect our children with the truth that they have been created for a higher purpose. As children receive care, they learn to value it. They will then grow up to be people who can move into the world, continuing to love and give care in their own spheres of influence. Entire societies and future generations will benefit when the lost art of caring is passionately celebrated and intentionally passed on.

TEN

THE REAL LIFE OF LOVE

Loving Jesus, Loving People

We must remember throughout our lives that in God's sight there are no little people and no little places. Only one thing is important: to be consecrated persons in God's place for us, at each moment. Those who think of themselves as little people in little places, if committed to Christ and living under his Lordship in the whole of life, may, by God's grace, change the flow of our generation.

—Francis Schaeffer, *No Little People*

In June of 1983 my mom was diagnosed with cancer. After a seven-month battle, and in spite of chemotherapy treatments, she died at home. During that seven-month period, my sister and I had many opportunities to give back to Mom a tiny portion of the nurturing and care she had given us. The most difficult but intensely intimate time was the last week of her life as we took care of her at home.

In the midst of losing our mother, a hospice nurse named Maddie came to encourage us and help my sister, stepfather, and me stay with Mom for the duration. Her death was painful, and it was terrifying for my sister Paula and me to watch her suffer. Several times we questioned if it was right to have her at home rather than in the hospital. But it's what she wanted, and Maddie's reassuring presence confirmed that we were doing the right thing. She showed us how to face death head-on, continuing to care for Mom's personal needs, doing everything we could to make her comfortable and being physically present with her. Maddie's knowledge of nurturing was profound. She reinforced what we sensed was true: that personal care and our physical presence were the very best gifts we could give. As our mother's bodily functions slipped away one by one, we tried to restore her physical dignity. Even as she slipped into a coma, we gave her bed baths, combed her hair, and trimmed and painted her fingernails and toenails. A well-kept appearance had always been important to Mom, and taking care of her body was the only way we had left to show our love.

Paula and I stayed up together for two nights in a row waiting for death to finish its work. We talked, prayed, read Scripture, and drank coffee to stay awake. We collapsed in tears when our strength and courage ran out. At one point in the vigil we baked cookies. We were desperate to do something normal during such an abnormal time.

In the early morning hours after the second night, Mom's heart and lungs slowed down and gradually came to a halt. Paula, my stepdad, Arnold, Maddie, and I were surrounding her on the bed, holding her hands as she departed.

I was a young mother and a new Christian at the time, just beginning to learn the ways of a caregiving life. Since then, I've seen again and again the importance of presence, of caring for the body and the physical environment, and of telling God's truths in combination with observable, concrete acts of care. Our human need is the same from birth through death: We long to experience embodied love. We yearn to be loved in tangible ways.

TO LOVE THE THINGS HE LOVES

The art of caregiving, as a lifestyle *and* a distinct vocation, is nothing less than the art of God. As our minds are renewed through the Scriptures and the work of the Spirit to treasure what God treasures, we will, by design, show forth the heart of God. God loves what he has created. He loves beauty and has given us a world brimming over with creative details—the sweet face of a pansy, the stripes on a zebra, the delicate patterns of a butterfly wing. He loves the people he's created, and he has shown us through the life, death, and resurrection of Jesus the extravagant, costly ways of love.

To recover the art of caregiving, we must set our hearts to love what God loves. With our feet planted firmly on the ground and our love rooted in the physical acts of care and nurture, we bear in mind the eternal value of our work. We are caring for people who have an eternal destination. Even the simplest gesture of giving a glass of water to a thirsty person has eternal meaning. When the tedium of caregiving weighs us down, this per-spective brings refreshment and the strength to persevere. As we serve one person at a time in life-giving ways, beginning at home and moving out from there, we are simultaneously offering a personal service to Christ. This is an incomprehensible mystery, but it is true. Caring in this way is what it means to offer real love in the midst of real life.

A caregiving life is one with a guiding purpose. It is intentional. It's also frustrating, full of failure, and ripe with the need for God's grace and the mercy of fresh starts. We are broken, sinful, yet redeemed people who are still very much in the process of having Christ formed in us. We have moments of glory when everything—our heart, mind, motivations, and actions—comes together and we get it right. But more often we stumble, lash out, fall down, and come to a new realization of our need for God's grace and the filling of his Holy Spirit.

Embracing the seasons of caregiving helps us seize the moment for what it is: a portion of time that is small when seen against the whole of life on earth and the vast expanse of eternity. Yet what great significance is found in a single opportunity to love someone in a way that can never be repeated.

The Shape of Love

We can choose to live for the glory of God in the details of our daily lives. We can spread the fragrance of Christ to others by reaching for excellence and beauty, mirroring his care for us by caring for others sacrificially and with concern for detail. People are served in unexplainable ways when all their senses are engaged: sight, sound, touch, smell, and taste. It is the details that cause us to feel cared for, that take us back in our memories to the caregivers of our past, that encourage us to pass on the touch of God in ways that others have never experienced.

My mother-in-law told me of a time when she wanted to make something special for her aunt's birthday, a woman who had spent her life caring for others. "She always had a little sweet after dinner, and I thought, 'She never has pie.' But baking pies was not at all what I did well. Still, I kept feeling a nudge to do it, so I tried—and I made the most beautiful banana cream pie ever! When Dad and I took it over, she looked shocked at first and then the tears started falling. I said, 'What's wrong, Aunt Olie?' She answered, 'I'm eighty-two years old today, and nobody has ever made me a pie.'"

Our effort to go the extra mile affirms the dignity and value of another human being. Love is incarnated, tangible, real. Just as God's personality is displayed in his creation and his care, so our personality is seen as we express God's love through the gifts he's given us for the common good.

First John 3:16 offers us a definition of love. "This is how we know what love is: Jesus Christ laid down his life for us. And we ought to lay down our lives for our brothers." For most of us, laying down our life will not happen with one grand act. Rather, it will consist of a thousand small turnings of our will from its natural self-absorption to the self-giving ways of God.

Without a vital, living relationship to Jesus, none of us can sustain a life of artful caring for long. The human heart is riddled with selfishness. As the Holy Spirit brings us to new depths of wanting to give ourselves away for Jesus' sake, the battle of our sin nature rages inside us telling us to hold back, stay safe, and keep a tight grip on our self-interests. We repeatedly come face to face with our utter dependence on God to transform us. We are drawn again to abide in Jesus, to learn from him, and to ask for creativity and strength to lay down our life for others, one person at a time.

When we care, we reflect the artistry of God. When we express his creativity, his love, and his compassion, we draw others to him—and we ourselves come to a deeper understanding of the artists he has created us to be.

NOTES

Chapter 1

1. David Westcott, *Work Well, Live Well: Rediscovering a Biblical View of Work* (London: Marshall Pickering, 1996), 188.
2. Sarah Baumgartner Thurow, "Playing Our Work: A Providential Understanding," *Regeneration Quarterly* 2 (winter 1996): 22.
3. Francis A. Schaeffer, *The Mark of the Christian* (Downers Grove, Ill.: InterVarsity, 1970), 22.
4. Leland Ryken, *Redeeming the Time: A Christian Approach to Work and Leisure* (Grand Rapids: Baker, 1995), 91.
5. Edith Schaeffer, *Hidden Art* (Wheaton, Ill.: Tyndale, 1971).

Chapter 2

1. Lee Hardy, *The Fabric of This World* (Grand Rapids: Eerdmans, 1990), 80. (See also Romans 1:6 and 2 Peter 1:10.)
2. Os Guinness, *The Call* (Nashville: Word, 1998), 4.
3. Guinness, *The Call,* 179.
4. Danielle Crittenden, *What Our Mothers Didn't Tell Us: Why Happiness Eludes the Modern Woman* (New York: Simon and Schuster, 1999), 97.
5. G. K. Chesterton, *What's Wrong with the World?* (San Francisco: Ignatius Press, 1994), 94.
6. Chesterton, *What's Wrong with the World?* 94-5.

Chapter 3

1. Edith Schaeffer, *Common Sense Christian Living* (Grand Rapids: Baker, 1983), 105.
2. Dorothy C. Bass, *Receiving the Day: Christian Practices for Opening the Gift of Time* (San Francisco: Jossey-Bass, 2000), 117-8.

Chapter 4

1. Christine D. Pohl, *Making Room: Recovering Hospitality as a Christian Tradition* (Grand Rapids: Eerdmans, 1999), x.

2. See also 1 Timothy 3:2; 1 Timothy 5:10; Titus 1:8; 1 Peter 4:9; and 3 John 8.

3. Glenna Matthews, *"Just a Housewife": The Rise and Fall of Domesticity in America* (New York: Oxford University Press, 1987), xiii.

4. Karen Burton Mains, *Open Heart, Open Home* (Wheaton, Ill.: Mainstay Church Resources, 1976), 29.

5. Mains, *Open Heart, Open Home,* 30.

6. Wendell Berry, *What Are People For?* (New York: North Point Press, 1990), 147.

7. Dallas Willard, *The Divine Conspiracy: Rediscovering Our Hidden Life in God* (San Francisco: HarperSanFrancisco, 1998), 205.

8. Ana Maria Pineda, "Hospitality," *Cross Point* 11 (summer 1998): 33.

9. Margaret Talbot, "Dial-A-Wife," *The New Yorker* (20 and 27 October 1997): 207.

10. Nadya Labi, "Burning Out at Nine?" *Time* (23 November 1998): 86.

11. Pohl, *Making Room,* 75.

12. Pohl, *Making Room,* 112.

13. J. R. R. Tolkien, *The Hobbit* (New York: Ballantine, 1966), 61.

Chapter 5

1. Dallas Willard, *The Spirit of the Disciplines: Understanding How God Changes Lives* (San Francisco: HarperCollins, 1988), 179.

2. Willard, *The Spirit of the Disciplines,* 180.

3. From the title of Mary Bray Pipher's book, *The Shelter of Each Other* (New York: Putnam, 1996).

4. Edith Schaeffer, *What Is a Family?* (Old Tappan, N.J.: Revell, 1975).

5. Nita Andrews, Bible study at Christ Community Church, Nashville, Tenn., 28 January 1999.

6. Linda Burton, "The Making of a Home" in *What's a Smart Woman Like You Doing at Home?* by Linda Burton, Janet Dittmer, and Cheri Loveless (Vienna, Va.: Mothers At Home, 1992), 76.

Chapter 6

1. Dallas Willard, *The Divine Conspiracy: Rediscovering Our Hidden Life in God* (San Francisco: HarperSanFrancisco, 1998), 193.
2. William Barclay, *The Letter to the Romans, Revised Edition,* The Daily Study Bible series (Philadelphia: Westminster, 1975), 157.
3. Willard, *The Divine Conspiracy,* 111.
4. Leland Ryken, *Redeeming the Time: A Christian Approach to Work and Leisure* (Grand Rapids: Baker, 1995), 11.
5. As quoted in *How Now Shall We Live?* by Charles Colson and Nancy Pearcey (Wheaton, Ill.: Tyndale, 1999), 388.
6. David Westcott, *Work Well, Live Well: Rediscovering a Biblical View of Work* (London: Marshall Pickering, 1996), 202.
7. Lee Hardy, *The Fabric of This World* (Grand Rapids: Eerdmans, 1990), 80.

Chapter 7

1. John R. W. Stott, *The Message of Galatians*, The Bible Speaks Today series (Downers Grove, Ill.: InterVarsity, 1988), 158.
2. Huntly Dent, *The Feast of Santa Fe* (New York: Fireside, 1993).

Chapter 8

1. Anne Morrow Lindbergh, *Gift from the Sea* (New York: Vintage, 1991), 124.
2. Os Guinness, *The Call* (Nashville: Word, 1998), 73-4.
3. Guinness, *The Call,* 177.
4. Anne Lamott, *Traveling Mercies* (New York: Pantheon, 1999), 151-2.

5. William Barclay, *The Gospel of Matthew, Volume 2, Revised Edition*, Daily Study Bible series (Philadelphia: Westminster, 1975), 325.

6. Barclay, *The Gospel of Matthew*, 325.

Chapter 9

1. Letter by John R. Sauer from Mill Valley, California, published in "From My Mail: Thoughts on Duty to Kids and Bosses," "Work and Family" column, Sue Shellenbarger, *Wall Street Journal*, date of publication unknown.

2. Jonathan Alter, "It's 4:00 P.M. Do You Know Where Your Children Are?" *Newsweek* (27 April 1998): 30-1.

3. Sylvia Ann Hewlett and Cornel West, *The War Against Parents* (New York: Houghton Mifflin, 1998), 49-50.

4. Ruth Haley Barton, *The Truths That Free Us: A Woman's Calling to Spiritual Transformation* (Colorado Springs: Shaw, 2002), 2.

5. Elizabeth Perle McKenna, *When Work Doesn't Work Anymore: Women, Work, and Identity* (New York: Delacorte, 1997), 87, 89.

6. *The Expositor's Bible Commentary* for Macintosh, Zondervan *Interactive* Ver. 3.6, Zondervan, Grand Rapids, 1999.

7. Dick Keyes, *Beyond Identity: Finding Your Self in the Image and Character of God* (Ann Arbor, Mich.: Servant, 1984), 217.

8. In a 1998 report, the median income of families with an at-home parent was $38,835, while the median income of a dual income family was $57,637. (Charmaine Yoest, "What Do Parents Want?" *The American Enterprise*, 9, no. 3 [May/June 1998]: 49.)

9. Mardi Keyes, L'Abri tape library, "The Women of Proverbs 31," no. 2225 (Michigan City, Ind.: Sound Word Associates, ndd). audiocassette.

10. Os Guinness, *The Call* (Nashville: Word, 1998), 141.

ABOUT THE AUTHOR

Andi Ashworth has partnered with her husband—award-winning writer, producer, and performer Charlie Peacock–Ashworth—in business and ministry for nearly twenty years. Together they operate a recording studio and music production company in a suburb of Nashville. They have also cofounded and led a hospitality and teaching ministry called the Art House. Andi has been deeply involved in the women's ministry of her church. She is currently studying at Covenant Theological Seminary through the Covenant *Access* Distance Education program. She and Charlie are the parents of two grown children. Visit Andi's Web site at www.andiashworth.com.